Moyamoya Disease - A Disease to Count On in Your Daily Practice

Edited by Vicente Vanaclocha

Published in London, United Kingdom

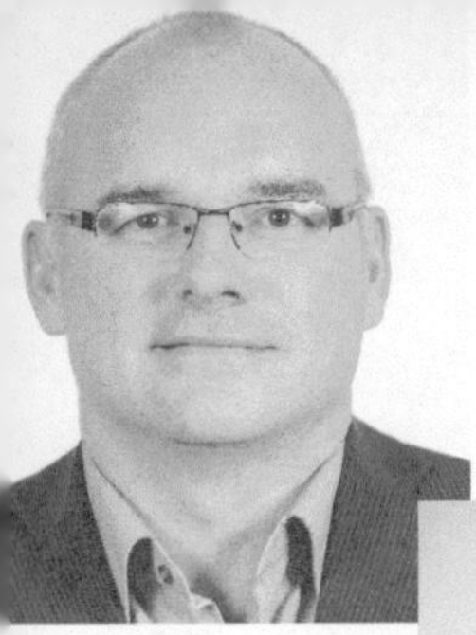
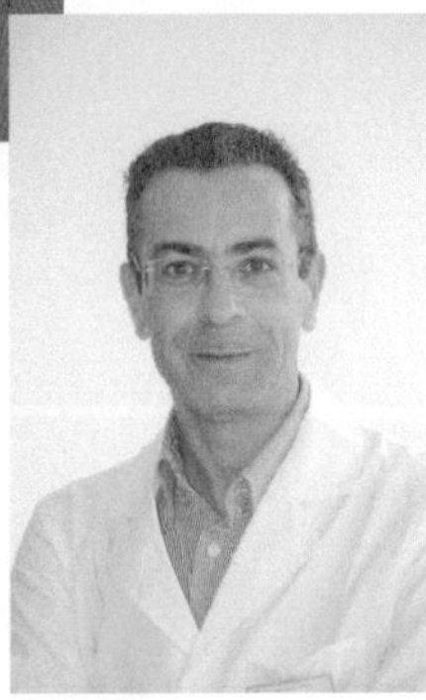
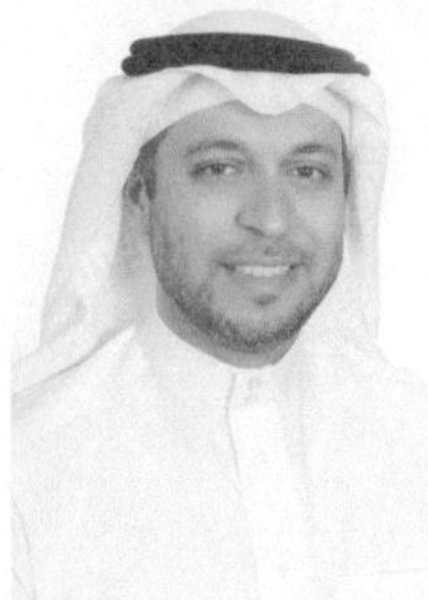
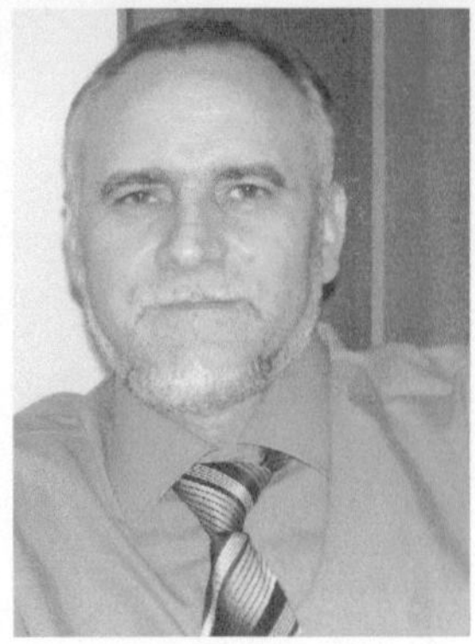
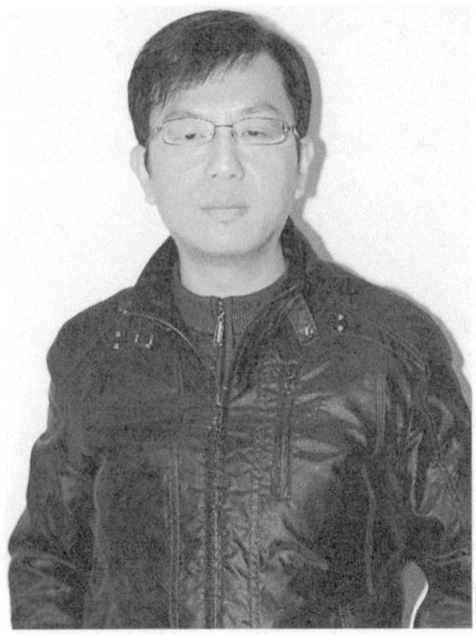
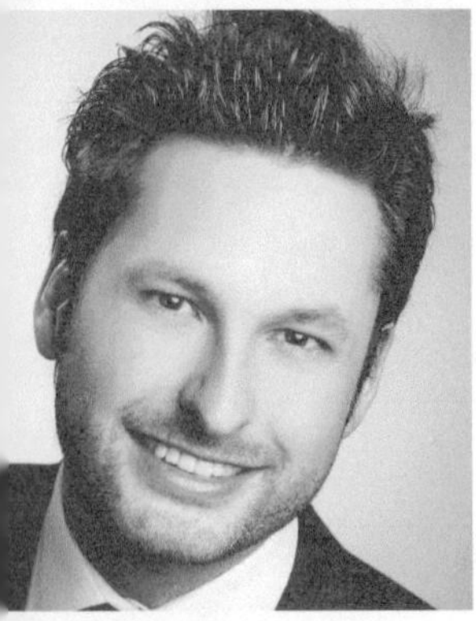
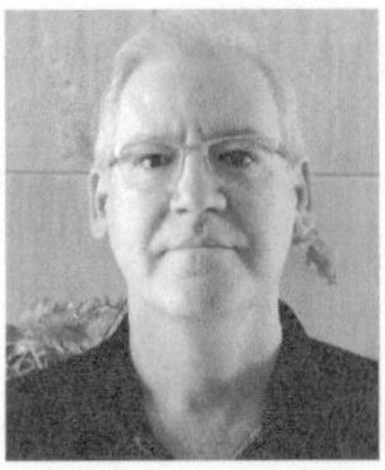

IntechOpen

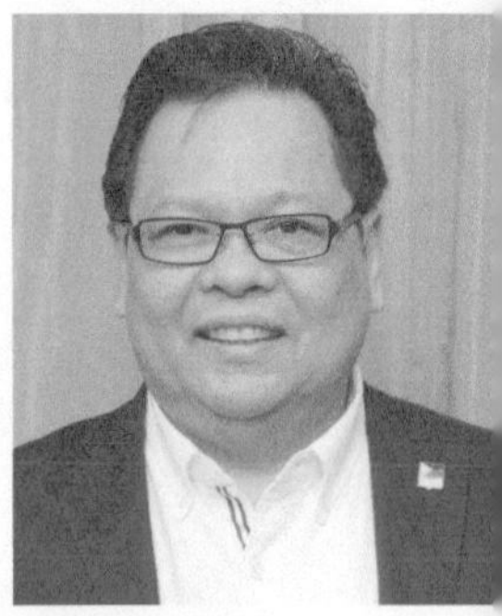
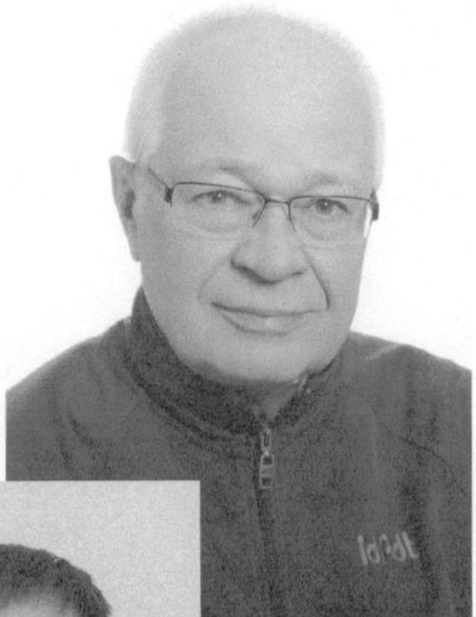
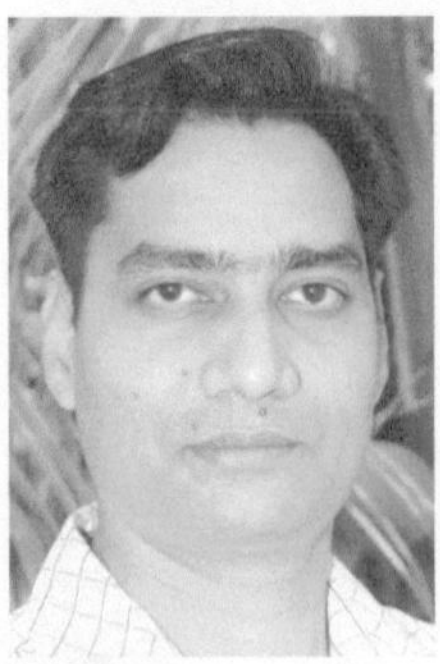
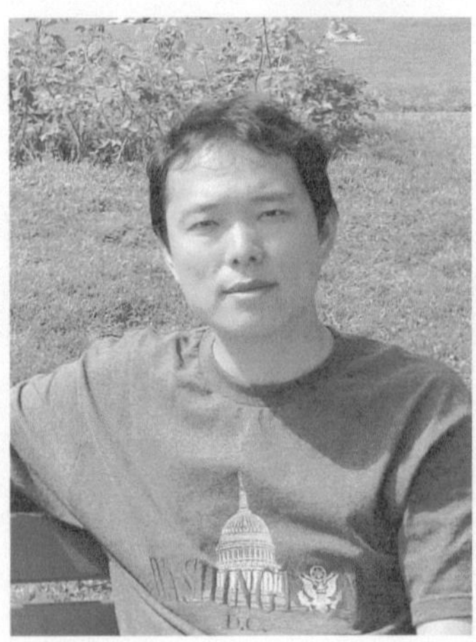
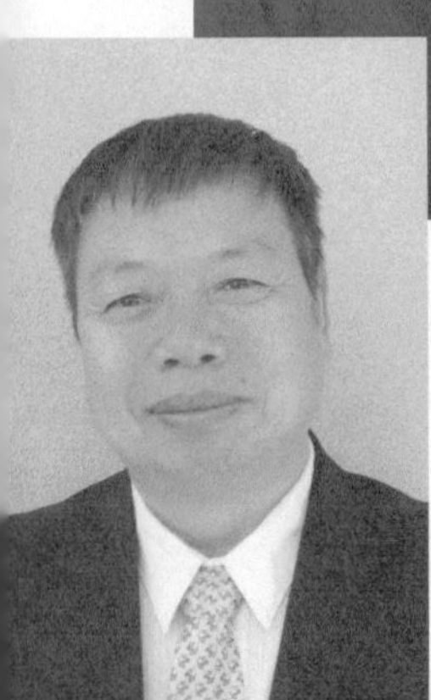
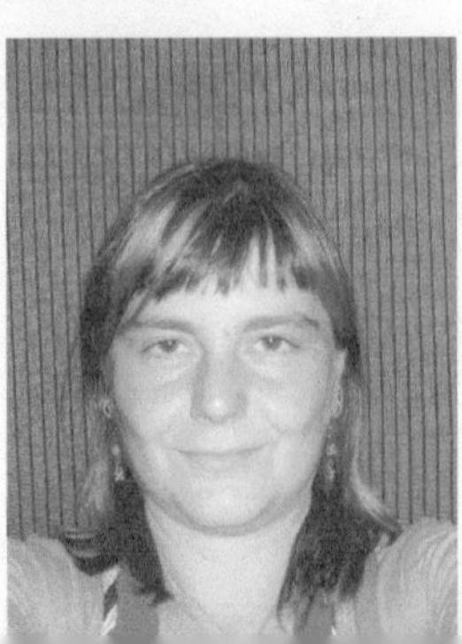

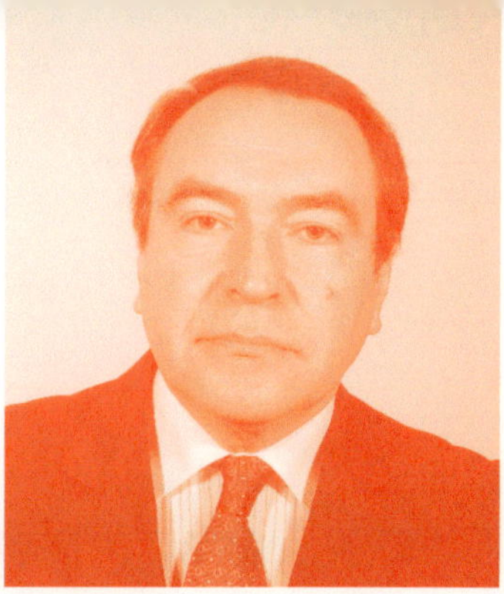
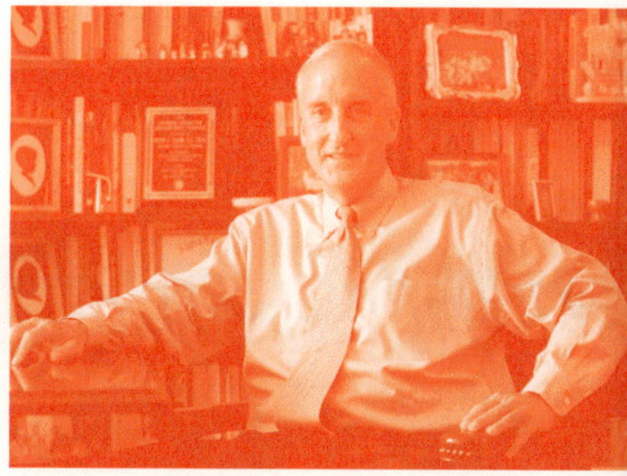
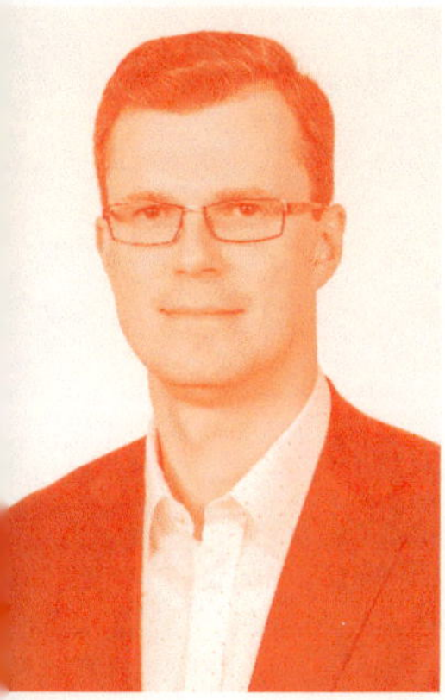
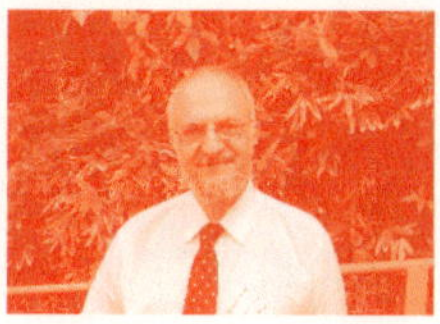
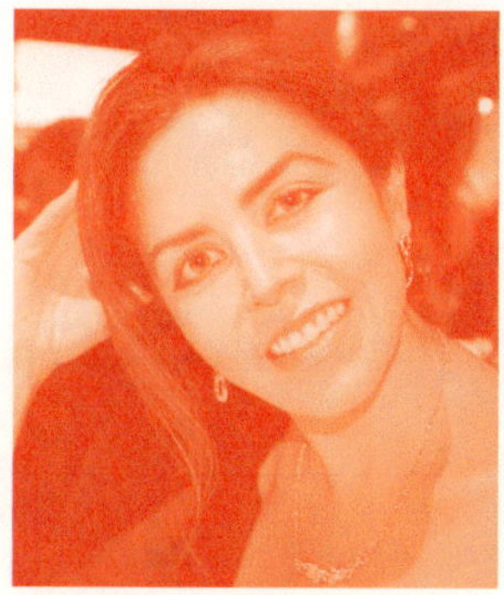

Supporting open minds since 2005

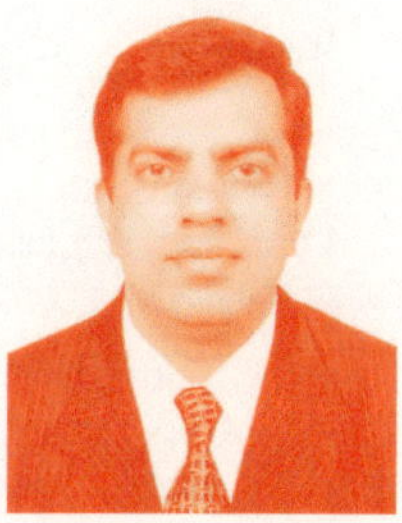
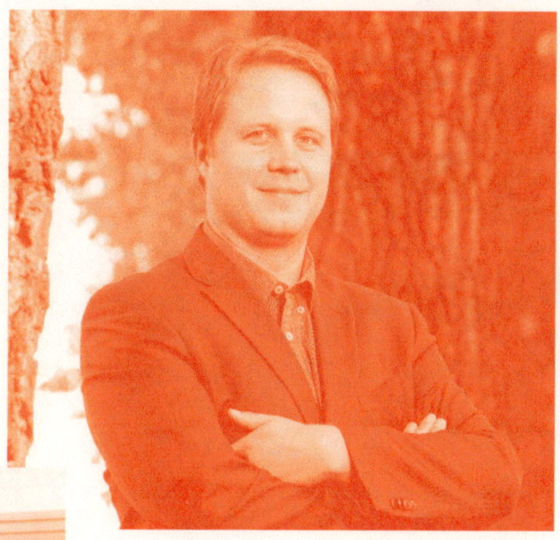
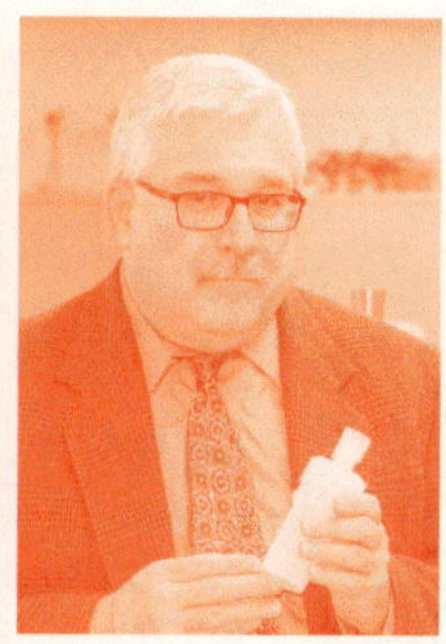
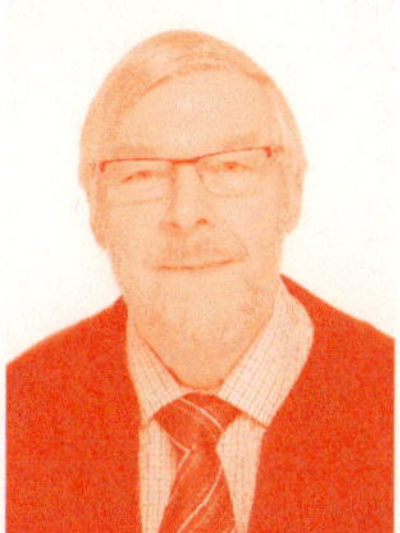
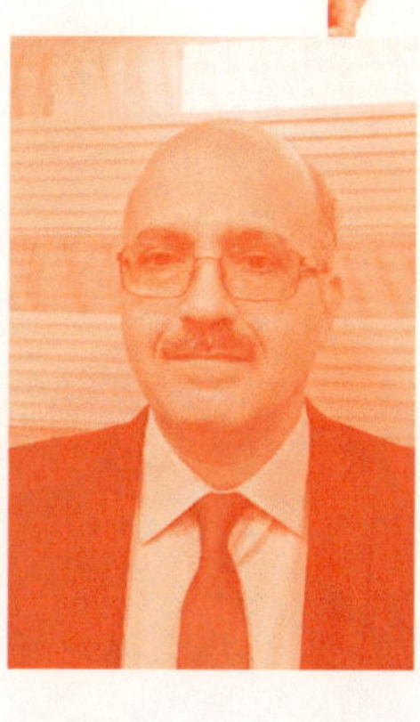
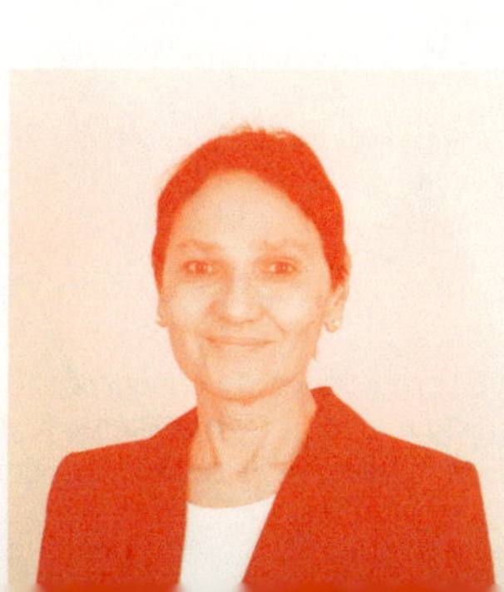
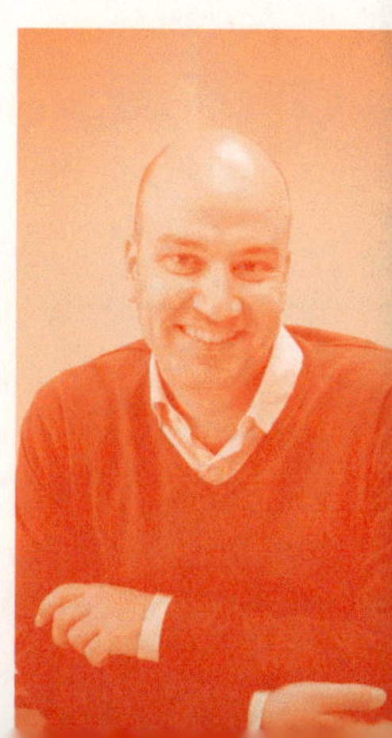

Moyamoya Disease - A Disease to Count On in Your Daily Practice
http://dx.doi.org/10.5772/intechopen.92950
Edited by Vicente Vanaclocha

Contributors
Sandhya Manorenj, Reshma Sultana Shaik, Man Mohan Mehndiratta, Ishu Goyal, Vasundhara Aggarwal, Natasha Gulati, Raúl Espert, Maria Engracia Gadea, Sombat Muengtaweepongsa, Sirinat Puengcharoen, Nattaphol Uransilp, Muhammad Jaffar Khan, Jazib Hassan, Sumayya Aboobacker, Mohamed El-Arref, Jafar Faraj, Tarek Tageldin, Vicente Vanaclocha, Nieves Saiz-Sapena, Leyre Vanaclocha

First published in London, United Kingdom, 2021 by IntechOpen
IntechOpen is the global imprint of INTECHOPEN LIMITED, registered in England and Wales, registration number: 11086078, 5 Princes Gate Court, London, SW7 2QJ, United Kingdom
Printed in Croatia

British Library Cataloguing-in-Publication Data
A catalogue record for this book is available from the British Library

Additional hard and PDF copies can be obtained from orders@intechopen.com

Moyamoya Disease - A Disease to Count On in Your Daily Practice
Edited by Vicente Vanaclocha
p. cm.
Print ISBN 978-1-83968-387-9
Online ISBN 978-1-83968-388-6
eBook (PDF) ISBN 978-1-83968-389-3

For EU product safety concerns:
IN TECH d.o.o., Prolaz Marije Krucifikse Kozulić 3, 51000 Rijeka, Croatia, info@intechopen.com or visit our website at intechopen.com.

Meet the editor

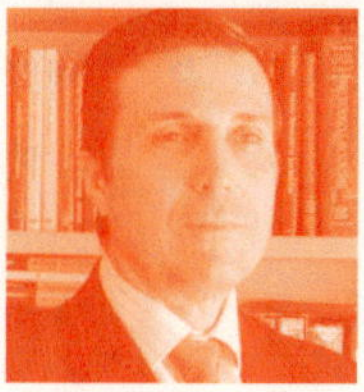

Professor Dr. Vicente Vanaclocha obtained his medical degree from the University of Valencia, Spain, and trained as a neurosurgeon in the university's affiliated hospital. He has placed great emphasis on training in his career, as evidenced by his fifteen long-term stays at various hospitals worldwide and his completion of 188 courses. He is always eager to learn and devoted to teaching. Dr. Vanaclocha has published eighty-two articles in peer-reviewed journals with close to 3,000 citations, eighteen book chapters, and three books. He has also been involved in humanitarian work in Syria and Egypt. He is a devoted husband and father of three lovely daughters.

Contents

Preface

Moyamoya disease is a progressive steno-occlusive process of the terminal internal carotid artery and its main branches with the development of an extensive network of collateral vessels, mainly at the lenticulostriate and choroidal arteries [1, 2]. This condition leads to ischemic and haemorrhagic strokes [3] and cognitive decline. Disease progression is the rule if left untreated [4].

Although it is more prevalent in East Asian countries [5, 6], it is commonly diagnosed in the USA [3] and Europe [7]. A chapter will deal with the differences in the regional prevalence of moyamoya disease. Moreover, its reported prevalence has been increasing over the years partly because of higher awareness in the medical profession, better diagnostic capacities [8, 9] and regular medical brain check-ups [4, 10]. As a result, the amount of asymptomatic patients diagnosed has rosed over time [11, 12]. The question is what to do with them because being asymptomatic today does not guarantee that they will remain so forever, nor will they have no silent brain infarctions or microbleeds [13].

Moreover, in this book, we will present evidence that these patients are not entirely asymptomatic. Instead, they suffer from a steadily progressing cognitive decline [14], particularly children [15–17]. Interestingly this cognitive decay seems to precede the onset of clinical symptoms due to haemorrhagic or ischemic strokes [14].

Surgical revascularization on asymptomatic moyamoya patients is controversial, particularly in children [18]. Although medical treatment with antithrombotic drugs is used for mild asymptomatic cases, their effectiveness is limited [5, 19]. A chapter in this book will enlighten on how to get the best of the moyamoya pharmacological treatment.

Direct, indirect or combined brain revascularization have shown better long-term results than conservative treatment [18, 20, 21], and a book chapter is devoted entirely to it.

Perioperative management must be exquisite to minimize morbidity and mortality. A chapter is presented by experienced colleagues that will enlighten the way we all must follow.

This book focuses on a disease uncommon in most world areas, stressing that perhaps it is not so uncommon because there are many, perhaps too many, asymptomatic or undiagnosed cases. And yet, we need to sharpen our clinical skills to diagnose the disease as early as possible and apply all the treatment options in due time and form. After all, this unforgiving condition will make patients pay a severe toll on sequelae and lost quality of life.

Vicente Vanaclocha
Professor,
Department of Surgery,
Division of Neurosurgery,
University of Valencia,
Valencia, Spain

References

[1] Suzuki J, Takaku A. Cerebrovascular «moyamoya» disease. Disease showing abnormal net-like vessels in base of brain. Arch Neurol. 1969;20(3):288-99.

[2] Suzuki J, Kodama N. Moyamoya disease--a review. Stroke. 1983;14(1):104-9.

[3] Uchino K, Johnston SC, Becker KJ, Tirschwell DL. Moyamoya disease in Washington State and California. Neurology. 2005;65(6):956-8.

[4] Jo K-I, Yeon JY, Hong S-C, Kim J-S. Clinical course of asymptomatic adult moyamoya disease. Cerebrovasc Dis Basel Switz. 2014;37(2):94-101.

[5] Shang S, Zhou D, Ya J, Li S, Yang Q, Ding Y, et al. Progress in moyamoya disease. Neurosurg Rev. 2020;43(2):371-82.

[6] Bao X-Y, Wang Q-N, Zhang Y, Zhang Q, Li D-S, Yang W-Z, et al. Epidemiology of Moyamoya Disease in China: Single-Center, Population-Based Study. World Neurosurg. 2019;122:e917-23.

[7] Yonekawa Y, Ogata N, Kaku Y, Taub E, Imhof HG. Moyamoya disease in Europe, past and present status. Clin Neurol Neurosurg. 1997;99 Suppl 2:S58-60.

[8] Ahn IM, Park D-H, Hann HJ, Kim KH, Kim HJ, Ahn HS. Incidence, prevalence, and survival of moyamoya disease in Korea: a nationwide, population-based study. Stroke. 2014;45(4):1090-5.

[9] Yang J, Hong JC, Oh CW, Kwon O-K, Hwang G, Kim JE, et al. Clinicoepidemiological features of asymptomatic moyamoya disease in adult patients. J Cerebrovasc Endovasc Neurosurg. 2014;16(3):241-6.

[10] Ikeda K, Iwasaki Y, Kashihara H, Hosozawa K-I, Anan K, Tamura M, et al. Adult moyamoya disease in the asymptomatic Japanese population. J Clin Neurosci Off J Neurosurg Soc Australas. 2006;13(3):334-8.

[11] Ryu GW, Yang YS, Choi M, Shim KW. Lived experiences of adult patients with moyamoya disease: A qualitative case study. Jpn J Nurs Sci JJNS. 2020;17(3):e12332.

[12] Luo R, Gao F, Deng X, Zhang D, Zhang Y. Results of Conservative Follow-up or Surgical Treatment of Moyamoya Patients Who Present without Hemorrhage, Transient Ischemic Attack, or Stroke. World Neurosurg. 2017;108:683-9.

[13] Kuroda S, AMORE Study Group. Asymptomatic moyamoya disease: literature review and ongoing AMORE study. Neurol Med Chir (Tokyo). 2015;55(3):194-8.

[14] He S, Duan R, Liu Z, Ye X, Yuan L, Li T, et al. Characteristics of cognitive impairment in adult asymptomatic moyamoya disease. BMC Neurol. 2020;20(1):322.

[15] Imaizumi T, Hayashi K, Saito K, Osawa M, Fukuyama Y. Long-term outcomes of pediatric moyamoya disease monitored to adulthood. Pediatr Neurol. 1998;18(4):321-5.

[16] Kurokawa T, Tomita S, Ueda K, Narazaki O, Hanai T, Hasuo K, et al. Prognosis of occlusive disease of the circle of Willis (moyamoya disease) in children. Pediatr Neurol. 1985;1(5):274-7.

[17] Imaizumi C, Imaizumi T, Osawa M, Fukuyama Y, Takeshita M. Serial intelligence test scores in pediatric moyamoya disease. Neuropediatrics. 1999;30(6):294-9.

[18] Zeng H, Guo Y, Li Y, Yu X, Yan F, Tan X, et al. Comparison of Operative and Conservative Treatment for Asymptomatic Moyamoya Disease: Preliminary Experience in Small Retrospective Series. World Neurosurg. 2021;146:e955-60.

[19] Ge P, Zhang Q, Ye X, Liu X, Deng X, Li H, et al. Long-Term Outcome After Conservative Treatment and Direct Bypass Surgery of Moyamoya Disease at Late Suzuki Stage. World Neurosurg. 2017;103:283-90.

[20] Kawaguchi S, Okuno S, Sakaki T. Effect of direct arterial bypass on the prevention of future stroke in patients with the hemorrhagic variety of moyamoya disease. J Neurosurg. 2000;93(3):397-401.

[21] Kuroda S, Houkin K, Ishikawa T, Nakayama N, Iwasaki Y. Novel bypass surgery for moyamoya disease using pericranial flap: its impacts on cerebral hemodynamics and long-term outcome. Neurosurgery. 2010;66(6):1093-101; discussion 1101.

Dedication

To my wife and daughters, the compass of my life, for their unconditional love and support.

Acknowledgments

I want to show my special gratitude to Dolores Kuzelj for her help and assistance.

Section 1

Introduction

Chapter 1

Introductory Chapter: Moyamoya Disease, Silent Killer

Vicente Vanaclocha, Nieves Saiz-Sapena and Leyre Vanaclocha

1. Introduction

Moyamoya disease is a cerebrovascular ailment that entails a progressive steno-occlusive process of the terminal internal carotid artery and its main branches. Secondarily it induces the development of an extensive network of unusual reticular collateral vessels at the skull base, mainly at the lenticulostriate and choroidal arteries [1–4]. These abnormal vessels create a hazy picture on cerebral angiogram that looks like a "puff of cigarette smoke drifting in the air" [5], which is the meaning of moyamoya in the Japanese language. These abnormal collateral vessels undergo pathological changes that lead to the appearance of haemorrhages [6].

Moyamoya disease leads to ischemic and haemorrhagic brain strokes and induces cognitive impairment [2, 7–9], partly due to the cerebrovascular insults [8], chronic brain hypoperfusion and white matter involvement [10]. The cognitive decline seems to be more severe in the haemorrhagic than in the ischemic type [11]. Disease progression is typical if left untreated [12].

Moyamoya disease aetiology is mostly unknown [13, 14], and without precise knowledge in this area, it is challenging to devise an effective treatment that prevents and cures this disease.

2. Disease incidence and prevalence

It is more prevalent in East Asian countries [15–17], namely Japan (10.3/100,000 people in 2006) [5], Korea (9.1/100,000 in 2008) [18] and China (3.92/100,000 in 2010) [19] than in the USA [20] and Europe [21].

Moyamoya incidence and prevalence have been increasing steadily over the years. In Japan the reported incidence rose from 0.35/100,00 in 1995 [16] to 0.54/100,000 in 2003 [5] and 0.94/100,000 in 2006 and the prevalence from 3.16/100,000 in 1995 [16], to 6.03/100,000 in 2003 [5] and 10.4/100,000 in 2006 [5], with a 1.8:1 female to male ratio [22] and a 10%-15% [5, 22, 23] familial cases. Another important aspect is that while the affected parents presented moyamoya related clinical symptoms at 22-36 years of age, their siblings showed the first symptoms when they were 5-11 years old [24]. In the USA [25] and Europe [21], the incidence in 10 times smaller, and the female to male ratio 2.2:1 [21]. In 2005 in the USA, the incidence was 0.086 cases/100,000 inhabitants [20].

Moyamoya disease has two peaks in incidence. The first in children before 18 years of age (maximum at 5-9 years old) and the second in adults in the fourth and fifth decades of life (highest rate from 35 to 45 years of age) [5, 17, 22, 26, 27]. In 47.8% of the patients, symptoms start before ten years of age [14].

IntechOpen

In Japan, the paediatric prevalence is the highest worldwide, with 3 cases per 100,000 children [5, 22, 28].

3. Asymptomatic moyamoya disease

It has been described as moyamoya features in the absence of any ischemic or haemorrhagic stroke [12]. The number of these patients has increased progressively over the years with improved diagnostic capacities [5, 24, 29–32] and the introduction of regular medical brain check-ups [12, 33]. In the Japan brain check-ups, the percentage of positive asymptomatic moyamoya patients was 0.07% (0.05% for males and 0.10% for females) with a female to male ratio of 3.3:1, mean age of 54 years [33]. Most of these asymptomatic patients were adults [34–37]. In children, the diagnosis can be unduly delayed due to their inability to communicate adequately, particularly at a very young ages [38].

But clinically asymptomatic patients do not mean that they have no pathological findings. In Japan, 20-30% of them harboured a cerebral infarction in watershed brain areas [24, 31] while the incidence of asymptomatic brain infarction in the general Japanese population in their fifth decade of life was 4.4% [39]. Additionally, 15-44% of adult moyamoya asymptomatic patients have clinically silent microbleeds [40–42] in the basal ganglia, thalamus and periventricular areas [43]. In a multicenter study in Japan, 34.3% of asymptomatic moyamoya patients with a normal cerebral blood flow had reduced cerebral vascular reserve [43]. In the follow-up, 12.5% [30] to 30% [12] of these patients suffered transitory ischemic attacks, ischemic or haemorrhagic stroke [12, 24, 31, 32], with a 3.2% annual stroke risk [12, 30, 31]. The female gender was associated with a greater risk of disease progression [31].

In Korea, the symptomatic progression in asymptomatic moyamoya patients was radiological in 12% and clinical in 5.3% with a reduced cerebral reserve capacity in 9.3% [30]. Clinical progression has been the rule worldwide for paediatric asymptomatic moyamoya patients [44]. As asymptomatic moyamoya disease is not a stable situation [12, 45, 46] close surveillance is mandatory, notably if there is a reduced cerebral vascular reserve [12, 30], ivy sign on MRI flair imaging [47, 48] or smoking habit [12]. The ivy sign is associated with an impaired cerebrovascular hemodynamic status [47]. It has been reported in 31.3% of asymptomatic moyamoya patients [47] that rises to 66% in those that already have ischemic stroke-related symptoms [48–50].

Moreover, these patients are not entirely asymptomatic but suffer from a steady cognitive decline in intelligence, spatial imagination, working memory, working memory-backwards digit span, computational ability, complex subtraction, complex arithmetic and word short-term memory [8, 51], particularly in children [45, 52, 53]. This cognitive decay precedes the onset of clinical symptoms due to brain infarction, or haemorrhage [8] and inevitable worsens when these cerebrovascular insults happen [51, 54]. Additionally, asymptomatic moyamoya patients can suffer from ischemic or haemorrhagic strokes [31]. Another critical aspect is that 20% of moyamoya children who undergo ischemic strokes are handicapped to undergo an independent social life [45, 53, 55].

Some have recommended performing surgical revascularization on asymptomatic moyamoya patients, particularly children, to prevent this unpleasant progressive neurological and cognitive deterioration [30, 44, 54]. Some have suggested undertaking surgical treatment if the ivy sign is seen in MRI flair imaging [47]. In any case, symptomatic progression in previously asymptomatic patients should be addressed with aggressive surgical revascularization in adults and children [30] as it halts disease progression [31].

4. Treatment modalities

Medical treatment with antithrombotic drugs (aspirin [56], cilostazol [57], clopidogrel [58, 59], low molecular-weight heparin, argatroban) [60] or calcium channel blockers [61] is used for mild asymptomatic cases, although their effectiveness has never been proven convincingly [15, 62]. Cilostazol is preferred over aspirin and clopidogrel because of its lower hemorrhagic risk [60], and clopidogrel recommended when aspirin is not tolerated [60]. These antithrombotic agents are advised for the ischemic-type moyamoya disease [15]. In any case, they are not very useful [63] as some researchers have reported an almost 3-fold chance of future neurological deterioration in the patients treated conservatively compared to those treated surgically [54, 64].

Direct, indirect or combined revascularization provides much better long-term results than conservative treatment, minimising the risk of ischemic and haemorrhagic strokes [54, 65, 66]. Early surgical intervention, particularly in paediatric patients, reduces cerebrovascular events and should be considered in asymptomatic children [44, 67]. Specific hospital perioperative morbidity and mortality have to be considered when recommending surgical treatment to these patients [12]. Thus, surgical treatment should be advised a soon as there is any sign of clinical or subclinical deterioration.

5. Conclusions

Moyamoya disease is more prevalent than previously thought because many patients go undiagnosed. Once diagnosed, asymptomatic patients may already harbour a cognitive decline long before cerebrovascular events take place. The only effective treatment is surgical revascularization, which should be undertaken as soon as any clinical deterioration sign occurs. Many posit that preventive surgical treatment should be recommended to asymptomatic patients, particularly in the paediatric age group.

Author details

Vicente Vanaclocha[1]*, Nieves Saiz-Sapena[2] and Leyre Vanaclocha[3]

1 University of Valencia, Spain

2 Hospital General Universitario de Valencia, Valencia, Spain

3 Medical School, University College London, London, United Kingdom

*Address all correspondence to: vvanaclo@hotmail.com

References

[1] Suzuki, J. & Takaku, A. Cerebrovascular 'moyamoya' disease. Disease showing abnormal net-like vessels in base of brain. Arch. Neurol. **20**, 288-299 (1969).

[2] Kuroda, S. & Houkin, K. Moyamoya disease: current concepts and future perspectives. Lancet Neurol. 7, 1056-1066 (2008).

[3] Suzuki, J. & Kodama, N. Moyamoya disease--a review. Stroke **14**, 104-109 (1983).

[4] Scott, R. M. & Smith, E. R. Moyamoya disease and moyamoya syndrome. N. Engl. J. Med. **360**, 1226-1237 (2009).

[5] Baba, T., Houkin, K. & Kuroda, S. Novel epidemiological features of moyamoya disease. J. Neurol. Neurosurg. Psychiatry **79**, 900-904 (2008).

[6] Funaki, T. *et al.* Effect of choroidal collateral vessels on de novo hemorrhage in moyamoya disease: analysis of nonhemorrhagic hemispheres in the Japan Adult Moyamoya Trial. J. Neurosurg. **132**, 408-414 (2019).

[7] Fang, L. *et al.* Different aspects of dysexecutive syndrome in patients with moyamoya disease and its clinical subtypes. J. Neurosurg. **125**, 299-307 (2016).

[8] He, S. *et al.* Characteristics of cognitive impairment in adult asymptomatic moyamoya disease. BMC Neurol. **20**, 322 (2020).

[9] Festa, J. R. *et al.* Neurocognitive dysfunction in adult moyamoya disease. J. Neurol. **257**, 806-815 (2010).

[10] Liu, Z. *et al.* Association between white matter impairment and cognitive dysfunction in patients with ischemic Moyamoya disease. BMC Neurol. **20**, 302 (2020).

[11] Su, S.-H., Hai, J., Zhang, L., Yu, F. & Wu, Y.-F. Assessment of cognitive function in adult patients with hemorrhagic moyamoya disease who received no surgical revascularization. Eur. J. Neurol. **20**, 1081-1087 (2013).

[12] Jo, K.-I., Yeon, J. Y., Hong, S.-C. & Kim, J.-S. Clinical course of asymptomatic adult moyamoya disease. Cerebrovasc. Dis. Basel Switz. **37**, 94-101 (2014).

[13] Mikami, T., Suzuki, H., Komatsu, K. & Mikuni, N. Influence of Inflammatory Disease on the Pathophysiology of Moyamoya Disease and Quasi-moyamoya Disease. Neurol. Med. Chir. (Tokyo) **59**, 361-370 (2019).

[14] Huang, S., Guo, Z.-N., Shi, M., Yang, Y. & Rao, M. Etiology and pathogenesis of Moyamoya Disease: An update on disease prevalence. Int. J. Stroke Off. J. Int. Stroke Soc. **12**, 246-253 (2017).

[15] Shang, S. *et al.* Progress in moyamoya disease. Neurosurg. Rev. **43**, 371-382 (2020).

[16] Ikezaki, K., Inamura, T., Kawano, T. & Fukui, M. Clinical features of probable moyamoya disease in Japan. Clin. Neurol. Neurosurg. **99 Suppl 2**, S173-S177 (1997).

[17] Bao, X.-Y. *et al.* Epidemiology of Moyamoya Disease in China: Single-Center, Population-Based Study. World Neurosurg. **122**, e917–e923 (2019).

[18] Im, S. H. *et al.* Prevalence and epidemiological features of moyamoya disease in Korea. J. Cerebrovasc. Endovasc. Neurosurg. **14**, 75-78 (2012).

[19] Miao, W. *et al.* Epidemiological and clinical features of Moyamoya disease in

Nanjing, China. *Clin. Neurol. Neurosurg.* **112**, 199-203 (2010).

[20] Uchino, K., Johnston, S. C., Becker, K. J. & Tirschwell, D. L. Moyamoya disease in Washington State and California. Neurology **65**, 956-958 (2005).

[21] Yonekawa, Y., Ogata, N., Kaku, Y., Taub, E. & Imhof, H. G. Moyamoya disease in Europe, past and present status. *Clin. Neurol. Neurosurg.* **99 Suppl 2**, S58-S60 (1997).

[22] Wakai, K. *et al.* Epidemiological features of moyamoya disease in Japan: findings from a nationwide survey. Clin. Neurol. Neurosurg. **99 Suppl** 2, S1-S5 (1997).

[23] Yamauchi, T., Houkin, K., Tada, M. & Abe, H. Familial occurrence of moyamoya disease. Clin. Neurol. Neurosurg. **99 Suppl** 2, S162-S167 (1997).

[24] Nanba, R. *et al.* [Clinical features and outcomes of 10 asymptomatic adult patients with moyamoya disease]. No Shinkei Geka. **31**, 1291-1295 (2003).

[25] Numaguchi, Y. *et al.* Moyamoya disease in the United States. Clin. Neurol. Neurosurg. **99 Suppl** 2, S26-S30 (1997).

[26] Fujimura, M., Bang, O. Y. & Kim, J. S. Moyamoya Disease. Front. Neurol. Neurosci. **40**, 204-220 (2016).

[27] Han, D. H. *et al.* A co-operative study: clinical characteristics of 334 Korean patients with moyamoya disease treated at neurosurgical institutes (1976-1994). The Korean Society for Cerebrovascular Disease. *Acta Neurochir. (Wien)* **142**, 1263-1273; discussion 1273-1274 (2000).

[28] Nagaraja, D., Verma, A., Taly, A. B., Kumar, M. V. & Jayakumar, P. N. Cerebrovascular disease in children. Acta Neurol. Scand. **90**, 251-255 (1994).

[29] Ahn, I. M. *et al.* Incidence, prevalence, and survival of moyamoya disease in Korea: a nationwide, population-based study. Stroke **45**, 1090-1095 (2014).

[30] Yang, J. *et al.* Clinicoepidemiological features of asymptomatic moyamoya disease in adult patients. J. Cerebrovasc. Endovasc. Neurosurg. **16**, 241-246 (2014).

[31] Kuroda, S., Hashimoto, N., Yoshimoto, T., Iwasaki, Y., & Research Committee on Moyamoya Disease in Japan. Radiological findings, clinical course, and outcome in asymptomatic moyamoya disease: results of multicenter survey in Japan. Stroke **38**, 1430-1435 (2007).

[32] Yamada, M., Fujii, K. & Fukui, M. [Clinical features and outcomes in patients with asymptomatic moyamoya disease--from the results of nation-wide questionnaire survey]. No Shinkei Geka. **33**, 337-342 (2005).

[33] Ikeda, K. *et al.* Adult moyamoya disease in the asymptomatic Japanese population. J. Clin. Neurosci. Off. J. Neurosurg. Soc. Australas. **13**, 334-338 (2006).

[34] Ryu, G. W., Yang, Y. S., Choi, M. & Shim, K. W. Lived experiences of adult patients with moyamoya disease: A qualitative case study. Jpn. J. Nurs. Sci. JJNS **17**, e12332 (2020).

[35] Luo, R., Gao, F., Deng, X., Zhang, D. & Zhang, Y. Results of Conservative Follow-up or Surgical Treatment of Moyamoya Patients Who Present without Hemorrhage, Transient Ischemic Attack, or Stroke. World Neurosurg. **108**, 683-689 (2017).

[36] Kleinloog, R., Regli, L., Rinkel, G. J. E. & Klijn, C. J. M. Regional differences

in incidence and patient characteristics of moyamoya disease: a systematic review. J. Neurol. Neurosurg. Psychiatry **83**, 531-536 (2012).

[37] Nariai, T. *et al.* Severe haemodynamic stress in selected subtypes of patients with moyamoya disease: a positron emission tomography study. J. Neurol. Neurosurg. Psychiatry **76**, 663-669 (2005).

[38] Jea, A., Smith, E. R., Robertson, R. & Scott, R. M. Moyamoya syndrome associated with Down syndrome: outcome after surgical revascularization. Pediatrics **116**, e694-e701 (2005).

[39] Shinkawa, A. *et al.* Silent cerebral infarction in a community-based autopsy series in Japan. The Hisayama Study. Stroke **26**, 380-385 (1995).

[40] Kuroda, S. & AMORE Study Group. Asymptomatic moyamoya disease: literature review and ongoing AMORE study. Neurol. Med. Chir. (Tokyo) **55**, 194-198 (2015).

[41] Ishikawa, T. *et al.* Prevalence of asymptomatic microbleeds in patients with moyamoya disease. *Neurol. Med. Chir. (Tokyo)* **45**, 495-500; discussion 500 (2005).

[42] Kikuta, K.-I. *et al.* Asymptomatic microbleeds in moyamoya disease: T2*-weighted gradient-echo magnetic resonance imaging study. J. Neurosurg. **102**, 470-475 (2005).

[43] Kuroda, S., Kashiwazaki, D., Ishikawa, T., Nakayama, N. & Houkin, K. Incidence, locations, and longitudinal course of silent microbleeds in moyamoya disease: a prospective T2*-weighted MRI study. Stroke **44**, 516-518 (2013).

[44] Lin, N. *et al.* Discovery of asymptomatic moyamoya arteriopathy in pediatric syndromic populations: radiographic and clinical progression. *Neurosurg.* Focus **31**, E6 (2011).

[45] Imaizumi, T., Hayashi, K., Saito, K., Osawa, M. & Fukuyama, Y. Long-term outcomes of pediatric moyamoya disease monitored to adulthood. Pediatr. Neurol. **18**, 321-325 (1998).

[46] Kuroda, S. *et al.* Incidence and clinical features of disease progression in adult moyamoya disease. Stroke **36**, 2148-2153 (2005).

[47] Vuignier, S. *et al.* Ivy sign, misery perfusion, and asymptomatic moyamoya disease: FLAIR imaging and (15)O-gas positron emission tomography. Acta Neurochir. (Wien) **155**, 2097-2104 (2013).

[48] Kawashima, M. *et al.* Unilateral hemispheric proliferation of ivy sign on fluid-attenuated inversion recovery images in moyamoya disease correlates highly with ipsilateral hemispheric decrease of cerebrovascular reserve. AJNR Am. J. Neuroradiol. **30**, 1709-1716 (2009).

[49] Fujiwara, H., Momoshima, S. & Kuribayashi, S. Leptomeningeal high signal intensity (ivy sign) on fluid-attenuated inversion-recovery (FLAIR) MR images in moyamoya disease. Eur. J. Radiol. **55**, 224-230 (2005).

[50] Yoon, H.-K., Shin, H.-J. & Chang, Y. W.' Ivy sign' in childhood moyamoya disease: depiction on FLAIR and contrast-enhanced T1-weighted MR images. Radiology **223**, 384-389 (2002).

[51] Karzmark, P., Zeifert, P. D., Bell-Stephens, T. E., Steinberg, G. K. & Dorfman, L. J. Neurocognitive impairment in adults with moyamoya disease without stroke. Neurosurgery **70**, 634-638 (2012).

[52] Kurokawa, T. *et al.* Prognosis of occlusive disease of the circle of Willis (moyamoya disease) in children. Pediatr. Neurol. **1**, 274-277 (1985).

[53] Imaizumi, C., Imaizumi, T., Osawa, M., Fukuyama, Y. & Takeshita, M. Serial intelligence test scores in pediatric moyamoya disease. Neuropediatrics **30**, 294-299 (1999).

[54] Zeng, H. *et al.* Comparison of Operative and Conservative Treatment for Asymptomatic Moyamoya Disease: Preliminary Experience in Small Retrospective Series. World Neurosurg. **146**, e955–e960 (2021).

[55] Matsushima, Y., Aoyagi, M., Masaoka, H., Suzuki, R. & Ohno, K. Mental outcome following encephaloduroarteriosynangiosis in children with moyamoya disease with the onset earlier than 5 years of age. Childs Nerv. Syst. ChNS Off. J. Int. Soc. Pediatr. Neurosurg. **6**, 440-443 (1990).

[56] Aihara, Y. *et al.* Aspirin use and platelet aggregation in ischemic onset-type pediatric moyamoya patients with intractable headaches (moya-ache). *Childs Nerv. Syst. ChNS Off. J. Int. Soc. Pediatr. Neurosurg.* (2021) doi:10.1007/s00381-020-04991-y.

[57] Ando, S. *et al.* Cilostazol may improve cognition better than clopidogrel in non-surgical adult patients with ischemic moyamoya disease: subanalysis of a prospective cohort. Neurol. Res. **41**, 480-487 (2019).

[58] Chiba, T. *et al.* Comparison of Effects between Clopidogrel and Cilostazol on Cerebral Perfusion in Nonsurgical Adult Patients with Symptomatically Ischemic Moyamoya Disease: Subanalysis of a Prospective Cohort. J. Stroke Cerebrovasc. Dis. Off. J. Natl. Stroke Assoc. **27**, 3373-3379 (2018).

[59] Soman, T. *et al.* The risks and safety of clopidogrel in pediatric arterial ischemic stroke. Stroke **37**, 1120-1122 (2006).

[60] Oki, K. *et al.* Trends of Antiplatelet Therapy for the Management of Moyamoya Disease in Japan: Results of a Nationwide Survey. J. Stroke Cerebrovasc. Dis. Off. J. Natl. Stroke Assoc. **27**, 3605-3612 (2018).

[61] Hosain, S. A., Hughes, J. T., Forem, S. L., Wisoff, J. & Fish, I. Use of a calcium channel blocker (nicardipine HCl) in the treatment of childhood moyamoya disease. J. Child Neurol. **9**, 378-380 (1994).

[62] Ge, P. *et al.* Long-Term Outcome After Conservative Treatment and Direct Bypass Surgery of Moyamoya Disease at Late Suzuki Stage. World Neurosurg. **103**, 283-290 (2017).

[63] Choi, J. U., Kim, D. S., Kim, E. Y. & Lee, K. C. Natural history of moyamoya disease: comparison of activity of daily living in surgery and non surgery groups. Clin. Neurol. Neurosurg. **99 Suppl 2**, S11-S18 (1997).

[64] Jang, D.-K. *et al.* Bypass surgery versus medical treatment for symptomatic moyamoya disease in adults. J. Neurosurg. **127**, 492-502 (2017).

[65] Kawaguchi, S., Okuno, S. & Sakaki, T. Effect of direct arterial bypass on the prevention of future stroke in patients with the hemorrhagic variety of moyamoya disease. J. Neurosurg. **93**, 397-401 (2000).

[66] Kuroda, S., Houkin, K., Ishikawa, T., Nakayama, N. & Iwasaki, Y. Novel bypass surgery for moyamoya disease using pericranial flap: its impacts on cerebral hemodynamics and long-term outcome. *Neurosurgery* **66**, 1093-1101; discussion 1101 (2010).

[67] Kim, S.-K. *et al.* Moyamoya disease among young patients: its aggressive clinical course and the role of active surgical treatment. *Neurosurgery* **54**, 840-844; discussion 844-846 (2004).

Section 2

Epidemiology of Moyamoya Disease

Chapter 2

Moyamoya Disease Worldwide-Global Burden East and West

Man Mohan Mehndiratta, Ishu Goyal, Vasundhara Aggarwal and Natasha Singh Gulati

Abstract

The Moyamoya disease [MMD] is a cereberovascular disorder characterized by progressive stenosis of intracranial internal carotid arteries and compensatory collateral formation at the base of the brain, mainly around the circle of Willis. When no particular associated risk factors can be identified, it is termed as Moyamoya disease. However, it may be associated with other neurological and extra- neurological disorders where it is termed as Moyamoya syndrome [MMS]. The condition is predominantly seen in East Asia and has bimodal age of distribution. The clinical manifestations are also age dependant with ischemia predominating in childhood and hemorrhagic manifestations being more common in adults. The pathogenesis is not entirely known, but genetic susceptibility is believed to be an important predisposing factor. The Suzuki staging system is most widely used for evaluation and staging of Moyamoya disease. The gold standard diagnostic modality is cerebral angiography but magnetic resonance imaging [MRA] has also been employed for diagnosis. Treatment is primarily surgical revascularization which is of 3 types: direct, indirect or combined revascularization. Although the role of revascularization surgery has been well established for ischemic MMD, the ideal surgical approach and the role of surgery in hemorrhagic MMD remains controversial.

Keywords: moyamoya disease, moyamoya syndrome, stroke, cerebral angiography, revascularization

1. Introduction

Moyamoya disease [MMD] is a form of chronic cerebrovascular occlusion characterized by occlusion of terminal internal carotid artery [ICA] along with a network of collateral vessels at the base of the brain. The disease was first brought to light by Takeuchi and Shimizu, where they described a young man with bilateral occlusion of ICA which was found to be due to congenital hypoplasia rather than atherosclerotic lesion [1]. Similar cases have been described in Japanese literature. After that, the condition came to be known by various names and the term 'spontaneous occlusion of the circle of Willis' by Kudo gained popularity [2]. The disease was finally coined '*moyamoya*' by Suzuki and Takaku based on the abnormal vascular network at the base of the brain that resembles 'vague or hazy puff of smoke' which is called *moyamoya* in Japanese [3].

This cerebral angiopathy is broadly termed 'moyamoya phenomenon' comprising of two nosological entities. The cerebrovascular syndrome is called 'Moyamoya syndrome' [MMS] when it is associated with neurological and extra neurological diseases like Neurofibromatosis 1 [NF1], Down syndrome, thyroid disease, cranial irradiation, sickle cell anemia, among other pathological conditions [4]. The Guidelines of the Research Committee on the Pathology and Treatment of Spontaneous Occlusion of Circle of Willis defined isolated moyamoya angiopathy as being idiopathic and called it 'Moyamoya disease' [5].

MMD is more common in Asian ethnicities as compared to the Western population [6]. The increased prevalence in Japan, Korea and other East Asian countries raised genetic predisposition to this condition. Subsequently, Kamada*et al.* identified a susceptibility gene, Ringin Protein 213 [RNF 213], and it was seen that this gene was positively associated with familial MMD [7]. Symptomatology of MMD varies according to the age group. Cerebral ischemia is more common in the pediatric than in the adult age group, whereas, the hemorrhagic type is more common in >40 years of age. Only one type predominates in a particular patient, but the symptoms are often recurrent. The disease diagnosis often rests upon angiography, and revascularization procedures are performed to avoid recurrence of symptoms. The lack of understanding of the exact pathophysiologic mechanism of MMD limits the development of treatments to prevent vascular damage.

2. Methods used

A literature search was conducted using PubMed. The keywords used were Moyamoya disease, Moyamoya syndrome, 'puff of smoke', Suzuki classification, angiography, revascularization procedures etc. Relevant articles were reviewed in detail. The search was filtered to include as many recent publications as possible. An effort was made to compile and highlight the key differences in the disease's clinical profile from East to West.

3. Epidemiology

For a very long time, Moyamoya disease was thought to be a disease of Asian lineage, but now it has been observed to be prevalent across the world in people with many ethnic backgrounds. MMD has been most extensively studied in Japan, where it is the most common pediatric cerebrovascular disease [8]. It shows a prominent East–West gradient, with a in East Asian countries ten times higher than the Western countries [9]. MMD is most frequently seen in Japan, with an incidence of 0.35–1.13/1,00,000/year and a prevalence of 3.16–10.5/1,00,000 [10]. In a study done in Hokkaido, Japan, 267 new cases were diagnosed between 2002–2006 [8]. The incidence and prevalence were also found to be high in other Asian countries like Korea, China and Taiwan [11]. The incidence in all these countries is found to be increasing over the years, most likely due to advancements in diagnostic modalities and a better understanding of the genetic factors linked to the disease [12]. Studies from outside Asia are very few. The incidence in Washington state and California was 0.086/1,00,000, but in them the incidence in Asian Americans was 4.6 times that of White [9]. In Europe, the incidence of MMD was 1/10th of that in Japan. North America's incidence was as low as 0.09/1,00,000 individuals, although an increasing trend is now being noted [13].

A similar bimodal age distribution is seen across the world, with the first peak occurring at 5–14 years in the pediatric population and around 4th decade in adulthood [5]. In Japan, family history is present in 10–15% of cases, and the risk of the disease in a family member is about 30–40 times higher than the general population. A familial predisposition was less commonly seen in European countries. In most countries, the disease was more frequently seen in females, with male to female ratio ranging from 1:1.8 to 1:2.2 [10, 14]. These epidemiological parameters remained constant from East to West as evident in the literature review from across the world by Kim et al. [6].

4. Pathology

The pathological features have been described based on autopsy findings of cases of MMD. The most common lesion is intracranial hemorrhage, which occurs in basal ganglia, thalamus, hypothalamus and brain stem. The intracranial hemorrhage may show intraventricular extension. Other findings are subarachnoid hemorrhage and small infarcts in the capsule- ganglionic area [14]. The main pathological findings according to the vessels involved are mentioned below.

a. *The Circle of Willis*: The distal ends of the internal carotid artery, Circle of Willis and its major branches are narrowed, tapered and often occluded. The occlusion is because of intimal thickening with marked attenuation of media. The intimal thickening is composed of smooth muscle cell proliferation rather than lipid and lipid-laden macrophages deposition, as seen in atherosclerosis [15].

b. *Perforating vessels*: The branches of Circle of Willis, anterior choroidal arteries, posterior cerebral arteries become dilated. Numerous dilated and tortuous vessels then originate from these arteries to penetrate the base of the brain. Aneurysm formation can also be seen. These small arteries can be enlarged with thin-walled or thick-walled with luminal stenosis [16].

c. *Leptomeningeal Vessels:* Angiographic findings in MMD reveal leptomeningeal anastomosis between the three main cerebral arteries and transdural anastomosis from external carotid arteries. These form the abnormal collateral circulation seen as the 'puff of smoke' [17].

d. *Other features:* Intracranial aneurysms, stenosis in extracranial arteries like carotid, renal, pulmonary arteries, etc.

Thus, the pathology of the disease can be viewed as ICA [Internal carotid artery] to ECA [External carotid artery] prism, where the contribution of ICA to cerebral blood supply gradually decreases, and the compensatory vascular network is formed which is predominantly fed by ECA.

5. Pathogenesis

The mechanisms leading to the above-mentioned pathology are not entirely known. It is not clear what leads to migration and proliferation of smooth muscle cells in the intima and leads to its thickening. Moreover, why this thickening happens only in the circle of Willis is unknown. Many features of the disease point towards a hereditary predisposition- high incidence in Japanese people, familial occurrence, association with other congenital disorders like sickle cell anemia, neurofibromatosis, Down syndrome, etc. A multifactorial mode of inheritance has been suggested. A possible linkage of the disease with markers located on chromosome 6, chromosome 17, chromosome 8q23 has been suggested [18–20]. Recently, a genetic locus in the Ring Finger Protein [RNF] 213 gene was also associated with MMD [7]. A higher carrier rate in Eastern Asia probably explains the higher prevalence of the disorder in Japan and other eastern Asian countries as compared to the Western world [21].

Moyamoya angiopathy has been identified with many genetic disorders like Neurofibromatosis 1, Noonan syndrome, Costello syndrome, Sickle cell disease, GUCY1A3 mutations, BRCC3/MTCP1 gene mutation, Down syndrome, Turner syndrome, etc. [19] Moyamoya disease associated with other familial or acquired conditions has also been termed as 'quasi-MMD'. It was noted that unilateral presentation was more common than bilateral and hemorrhagic manifestations were less common in quasi- MMD [21].

Although genetic predisposition to the disease exists, the majority of cases are sporadic. Certain acquired factors have been suggested for disease progression. These include vasculitis [3], infections [20], cranial trauma [22], post-irradiation state [23] to name a few.

6. Clinical features

The pathological changes in cerebral arteries lead to cerebrovascular events in Moyamoya disease. Two peaks have been identified, at around ten years and 30–40 years. The peak occurs later in women than in men [24].

The symptoms can be classified in the following four main heads (**Figure 1**) [13].

Transient ischemic attacks [TIA] and infarct may present as a variety of symptoms- motor paresis, sensory disturbance, speech disturbances, alteration of consciousness [25]. Whereas these symptoms present acutely, mental decline, dyskinesias tend to progress over the years. Dilated collateral vessels in basal ganglia have been implicated in the development of choreiform movements [26]. Bilateral disease is associated with cognitive deficits. Hemorrhagic type is more common in adults >40 years of age and most commonly present with impaired consciousness. Irrespective of the primary pathology [ischemic/hemorrhagic], the symptoms tend to be recurrent and usually a single pathology predominates in each individual. Headache is another common symptom generally seen in children <14 years old [27]. Dilated transdural collaterals stimulate dural nociceptors precipitating migraine-like headaches. Headache may also be a manifestation of chronic hypoxemia.

The symptoms are triggered by hyperventilation, such as blowing/crying due to decreased cerebral blood flow secondary to CO_2 washout. Worsening is also seen

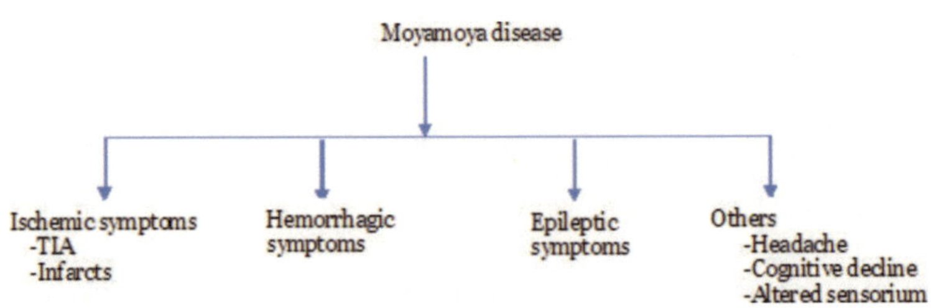

Figure 1.
Clinical symptoms of Moyamoya disease.

with infection of the upper respiratory tract. Hypertension and aging often contribute to hemorrhage, which may occur at repetitive intervals. Massive bleeding may even lead to death. Epilepsy, as a manifestation of the disease, is usually seen in children less than ten years of age [28].

The clinical features also tend to vary from East to West. The ischemic manifestations are more predominant in the US [United States] than in other eastern countries. The rate of hemorrhagic disease in adults in Asian countries is higher [42%] than in those of Asian descent residing in the US [29]. The disorder's overall spectrum remains constant worldwide, with ischemic manifestations as the main presenting feature in children and both ischemia and hemorrhage in adults.

7. Diagnosis

7.1 Angiography

Angiography is the gold standard for diagnosis and assessing disease progression. The hallmark findings of cerebral angiography are occlusion of intracranial internal carotid arteries (**Figure 2**) and abnormal smog-like arteriolar network [moyamoya vessels] at the base of the brain (**Figure 3**). The Circle of Willis and its main branches, leptomeningeal vessels and transdural anastomosis between ophthalmic artery, external carotid artery and vertebral artery are frequently seen. Involvement of posterior circulation is less commonly observed.

Suzuki et al. staged the disease progression into the following stages based on the angiographic findings [3, 22, 27].

1. Narrowing of the carotid forks

2. Initiation of moyamoya[dilated major cerebral artery and a slight network of collaterals]

3. Intensification of moyamoya with the disappearance of middle and anterior cerebral arteries

4. Minimization of moyamoya [disappearance of posterior cerebral artery and narrowing of individual moyamoya vessels]

5. Reduction of moyamoya [disappearance of main cerebral arteries, further minimization of moyamoya, increase in collaterals from external carotid arteries]

6. Disappearance of moyamoya [complete disappearance of moyamoya with blood flow derived only from the external carotid artery and vertebrobasilar system]

Apart from these changes, aneurysm formation can also be seen in angiography. A revised version of Suzuki staging system was given by Mugikura et al. (**Table 1**), where staging is done based on angiographic severity of stenosis of the middle cerebral artery and anterior cerebral artery [30].

Both the staging systems highlight that with the progression of the disease, the contribution of blood supply from ICA decreases and an intricate collateral network is formed which derives its blood flow from vessels outside the cerebral circulation.

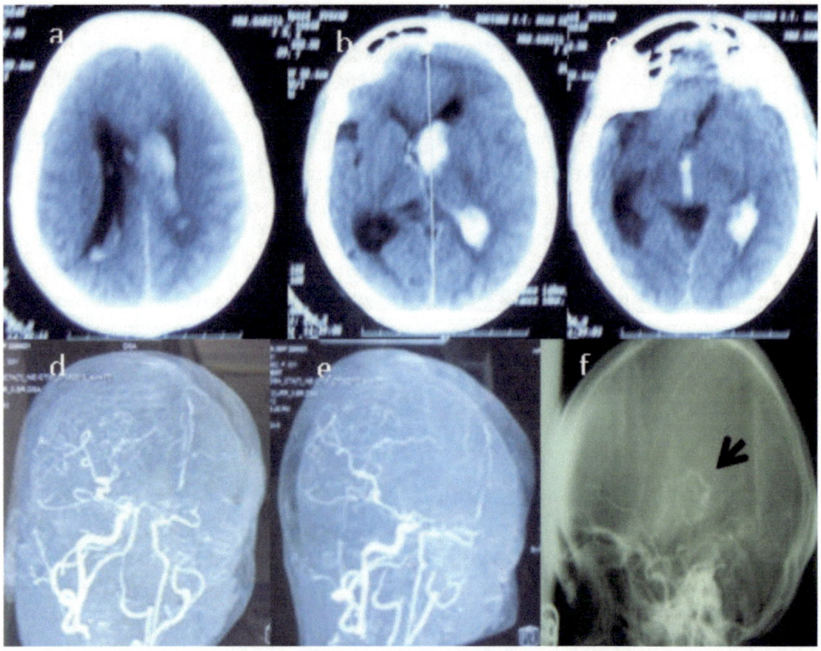

Figure 2.
Neuroimaging of a 40 years old lady who presented with ICH. Non-contrast CT axial sections of brain (a, b, c) show intraventricular hemorrhage involving bilateral lateral ventricles (L > R), third and fourth ventricle. Angiographic images (d, e) show occlusion of the supraclinoid segment of the left internal carotid artery and attenuation on the right side with lenticulostriate collaterals showing a "puff of smoke" appearance (f).

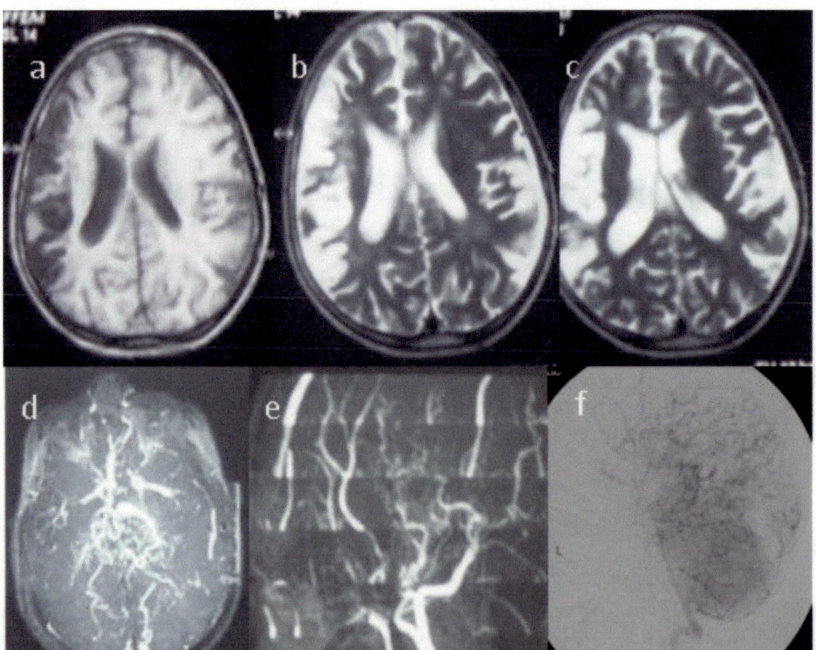

Figure 3.
Neuroimaging of a young boy of 6 years of age who presented with recurrent ischemic strokes. MRI brain axial sections show altered signal intensity areas hypointense on T1 (a) and hyperintense on T2 (b, c)) in bilateral frontoparietal cortex involving the MCA territory. Angiographic images show multiple tortuous collaterals involving both anterior (d) and posterior circulation (d, e, f) giving the typical **"puff of smoke"** *appearance on cerebral DSA (f).*

ICA Stage	Angiographic findings
I	Mild to moderate stenosis around carotid bifurcation, absent/slightly developed moyamoya, ACA/MCA branches opacified in anterograde fashion
II	Severe stenosis around carotid bifurcation, well developed moyamoya, several of ACA/MCA branches opacified in anterograde fashion
III	Occlusion of proximal ACA/MCA, well developed moyamoya, only a few of ACA/MCA branches are faintly opacified in anterograde fashion through the mesh work of ICA moyamoya
IV	Complete occlusion of proximal ACA and MCA, small amount of moyamoya, no opacification of either ACA/MCA branches in anterograde fashion
ACA- anterior cerebral artery, MCA- middle cerebral artery, ICA- internal cerebral artery.	

Table 1.
The angiographic ICA staging system modified by Mugikura et al.

7.2 Computed tomography [CT]

CT scan shows hyperdensities in basal ganglia, thalamus, ventricular system and subarachnoid spaces in the hemorrhagic type of MMD. In the ischemic type of the disease, lacunar infarcts can be seen as the areas of hypodensities. When contrast-enhanced, tortuous and curvilinear vessels in basal ganglia can be visualized which represent the moyamoya vessels.

Magnetic Resonance Imaging and Angiography [MRI and MRA].

MRI and MRA provide visualization of the arterial tree without being invasive as conventional angiography. In addition to this, MRI also helps demonstrate small

Score for each artery	MRA finding
Internal cerebral artery	
0	Normal
1	Stenosis of C1
2	Discontinuity of the C1 signal
3	Invisible
Middle cerebral artery	
0	Normal
1	Stenosis of M1
2	Discontinuity of the M1 signal
3	Invisible
Anterior cerebral artery	
0	Normal A2 and blood vessels distal to A2
1	Signal decrease A2 and its distal blood vessels
2	Invisible
Posterior cerebral arteries	
0	Normal P2 and blood vessels distal to P2
1	Signal decrease P2 and its distal blood vessels
2	Invisible

Table 2.
The classification and scoring based on the MRA findings- Score of each artery.

MRA total score	MRA stage
0–1	1
2–4	2
5–7	3
8–10	4

MRA: Magnetic Resonance Imaging.

Table 3.
The classification and scoring based on the MRA findings – MRA total Score.

subcortical lesions that are difficult to identify on the CT scan. MRA helps to identify the stenotic distal end of the internal carotid artery, small moyamoya vessels and dural anastomosis between external carotid arteries and vessels of the posterior circulation.

The classification and scoring based on the MRA findings are given above in **Tables 2** and **3**. This MRA scoring system also finds its place in the 2012 Guidelines for the Diagnosis and Treatment of MMD in Japan [5].

7.3 Ultrasonography

In patients with moyamoya disease, the involvement of many extracranial arteries like external carotid arteries, aorta, pulmonary artery, celiac artery, and renal artery has been described. Characteristic signs like ' champagne bottleneck sign' seen due to reduction in the diameter of proximal ICA and 'diamond reversal sign' due to smaller ICA diameter compared to external carotid artery have been demonstrated [31].

Though all the diagnostic modalities contribute to identifying and staging abnormal vasculature, angiography remains the mainstay of diagnosis. It is also helpful in documenting the postoperative resolution of moyamoya.

Electroencephalography [EEG].

The following EEG findings have been seen in moyamoya disease [32]:

1. Diffuse, bilateral, low voltage, slow spike and wave

2. 'Buildup' phenomenon- a diffuse pattern of slow waves

3. 'Rebuildup' phenomenon- diffuse slow waves during hyperventilation. This rebuild up phenomenon is seen due to decreased pCO2 on hyperventilation leading to cerebral ischemia and vasoconstriction.

8. Diagnostic guidelines

The advancements in various diagnostic modalities lead to the formulation of diagnostic guidelines for Moyamoya disease shown in **Table 4** [5].

8.1 Treatment

Moyamoya disease is a chronic progressive disease described earlier, leading to recurrent strokes due to internal carotid artery occlusion and ischemia due to narrow, low caliber collaterals. The illness's mainstay is revascularization surgery

A. Cerebral angiography should present at least the following findings:
1. Stenosis/occlusion at the terminal portion of ICA and/or at the proximal portion of ACA and/or MCA
2. Abnormal vascular network in the vicinity of stenotic/occluded vessels
3. Bilateral findings
B. Conventional angiogram not required when MRI/MRA demonstrate following findings:1.
1. Stenosis/occlusion at the terminal portion of ICA and/or at the proximal portion of ACA and/or MCA on MRA
2. Abnormal vascular network in the basal ganglia on MRA [>2 flow voids in basal ganglia in MRI].
3. Bilateral findings
C. Absence of arteriosclerosis, autoimmune disease, meningitis, brain neoplasm, down syndrome, Recklinghausen's disease, head trauma, irradiation to head, others.
D. Pathological findings:
1. Stenosis/occlusion due to intimal thickening at the terminal ICA, usually on both sides
2. Arteries of Circle of Willis show varying degree of stenosis/occlusion of intima, attenuation of media and waving of internal elastic lamina
3. Numerous small vascular channels around the Circle of Willis
4. Reticular conglomerates of small vessels in pia matter.
Definitive case: A/B + C[In children, a case that fulfills A1 and A2 or B1 and B2 on one side and remarkable stenosis of terminal ICA on opposite side is also included.]
Probable case: A1 and A2 [or B1 and B2] and C [unilateral]

Table 4.
Diagnostic guidelines for Moyamoya disease.

to increase the intracranial blood flow using extracerebral blood vessels by direct bypass or pialsynangiosis. The decision for surgical intervention is based on the patient's age, symptomatic/asymptomatic disease, ischemic/hemorrhagic manifestations, presence/absence of aneurysm and risk of recurrence.

The indication of surgery can be briefly summarized as follows in **Figure 4** [33].

8.2 Risk factors for disease recurrence

Moyamoya disease is known to progress over the years. The disease progression rate was reported to be approximately 20% over six years in those managed conservatively [34]. The risk factors of disease progression and subsequent ischemic stroke were identified as follows:

1. Female gender
2. Graves' disease
3. RNF213 variant
4. Family history positive [35]
5. Posterior circulation was also recognized as a decisive risk factor for ischemic stroke [36].

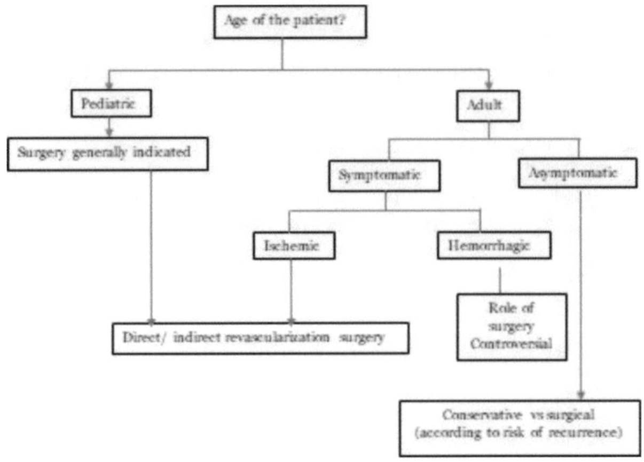

Figure 4.
Overview of the management of Moyamoya disease.

Moyamoya disease is a progressive disease, and symptomatic progression is seen in approximately two-thirds of patients [29]. In a large meta-analysis, where 1,156 people were studied, it was seen that 87% of those who underwent surgical revascularization showed partial or complete resolution of symptomatic cerebral ischemia [37].

A careful choice of treatment, that is, conservative vs. surgical should thus be made keeping in mind the above-mentioned risk factors.

8.3 Conservative treatment of mmd

The predominant manifestation of MMD is ischemic stroke. However, antiplatelet therapy is ineffective to prevent recurrent cerebral infarction in ischemic MMD. The ischemic insult in MMD patients is a consequence of hemodynamic instability. There is no evidence of endothelial dysfunction at the site of internal carotid artery bifurcation. Therefore, increased platelet adhesion is not seen in MMD. Hence, theoretically, antiplatelet drugs are ineffective for preventing ischemic stroke in MMD. Moreover, increased risk of hemorrhage remains with antiplatelets in patients with MMD [38]. The annual stroke rate in patients managed conservatively is between 3.2%–15% [35].

8.4 Indication of surgical revascularization

Surgical revascularization is done to increase the cerebral blood flow and restore reserve capacity. The increase in cerebral blood flow prevents recurrent cerebral infarction. The indications for surgical revascularization are:

1. Recurrent clinical symptoms due to cerebral ischemia

2. Pediatric MMD because pediatric MMD is more progressive than adult MMD. Early diagnosis and intervention are of paramount importance to prevent irreversible damage. In a recent study, Rosi et al. confirmed a high benefit/risk ratio, with better postoperative functional status and low rates for the need of surgical retreatment in the pediatric population undergoing surgical revascularization [39].

3. Role of revascularization surgery in asymptomatic MMD with stable hemodynamics is not well established but preferred by neurosurgeons given the disease

being a progressive disorder. Risk–benefit ratio determines the feasibility of the surgical intervention in such patients.

4. Role of revascularization surgery in hemorrhagic stroke is controversial.

With increased understanding of MMD being familial in at least some of the world's regions, it is being suggested that asymptomatic siblings and family members should be screened for moyamoya pathology. Whenever such a condition is detected, it should be managed surgically, keeping in mind the illness's progressive nature.

8.5 Surgical modalities for revascularization

8.5.1 Direct revascularization

Anastomosis is formed between the superficial temporal artery and cortical branches of middle cerebral arteries in this procedure. For posterior circulation, the occipital artery is used as a donor for nteroposterior cerebral arteries' cortical branches. The transdural or transcalvarial collateral channels should be preserved during the surgery.

The advantage of this procedure is an immediate improvement in the cerebral blood flow after surgery. However, the successful restoration of cerebral blood flow is operator dependant as it is challenging to perform. Moreover, postoperative hyperperfusion syndrome may develop after surgery leading to neurological deterioration. Patency and amount of bypass flow may be assessed postoperatively by digital subtraction angiography or quantitative magnetic resonance angiography.

The annual stroke rate after direct revascularization was reportedly 0–1.6% [40].

8.5.2 Indirect revascularization

The various surgical procedures are

1. Encephalomyosynangiosis[EMS] where deep temporal artery supplying the temporalis muscle is the vessel for neovascularization

2. Encephalo-duro-arteriosynangiosis[EDAS]: Here, superficial temporal artery[STA] is harvested with surrounding galea and periosteum; STA flap is placed with a galea cuff. The dura and galea are then sutured to cover the brain with arterial flap.

3. Encephalo-myo-arteriosynangiosis[EDAMS]

4. Encephalo-galeo-synangiosis[EGS]

5. Omental flap surgery

6. Multiple burr hole surgery

The last two surgeries are performed as primary or after failed revascularization by other techniques.

Indirect revascularization is relatively easier to perform than direct surgeries, and the incidence of hyperperfusion is also less. However, the improvement in cerebral revascularization takes longer than the direct surgeries where the effect is immediate.

After indirect revascularization, patients experienced 0–14.3% postoperative annual stroke rate [41].

Thus either of the indirect and direct revascularization procedures can be performed to rectify the underlying pathology, but the risk of recurrence is much less with the direct revascularization surgeries without any delay to the benefit.

8.6 Peri/postoperative complications

The following complications have been noted in the peri/postoperative period in MMD:

1. The risk of postoperative stroke has been estimated to be 1.6%- 16% [42].

2. The risk of perioperative ischemic complications is more in patients with unstable hemodynamics and advanced Suzuki stage with a lower cerebral blood flow.

3. Hemorrhagic stroke develops in 0.7%–8% [42].

4. Hyperperfusion syndrome- due to the chronic changes in cerebral blood vessels, the auto-regulatory function is lost, and the vascular reserve is decreased. The excessive blood flow immediately after the surgery is sometimes not well tolerated, leading to cerebral hemorrhage. Another factor that may predispose to intracranial hemorrhage is increased vascular permeability secondary to chronic ischemia.

5. Epidural hematoma mainly in the pediatric population.

6. Skin problems due to scalp ischemia after revascularization.

9. Conclusion

Moyamoya disease is a chronic progressive vasculopathy seen in children and adults, characterized by occlusion/stenosis at the terminal portions of the internal carotid artery and abnormal collateral network formation at the base of the brain. It is predominantly seen in Asian countries. It may be idiopathic [moyamoya disease] or associated with other disorders when it is called moyamoya syndrome. Various angiographic and magnetic resonance angiographic findings have been described which form the basis of the diagnostic guidelines for MMD. It may present as an ischemic/hemorrhagic stroke. It is generally managed with direct/indirect revascularization surgical techniques that aim to restore the cerebral blood flow and prevent strokes that restore the cerebral blood flow and prevent strokes' recurrence.

Author details

Man Mohan Mehndiratta[1,2]*, Ishu Goyal[3], Vasundhara Aggarwal[3] and Natasha Singh Gulati[3]

1 Department of Neurology, B.L. Kapur Hospital (Max Health Care Group), Centre for Neurosciences, New Delhi, India

2 Department of Neurology, Janakpuri Super Specialty Hospital, Janakpuri, New Delhi, India

3 Janakpuri Super Specialty Hospital Society, New Delhi, India

*Address all correspondence to: mmehndi@hotmail.com

References

[1] Smith JL. Understanding and treating moyamoya disease in children. Neurosurg Focus. 2009 Apr;26(4): E4. doi: 10.3171/2000.01.FOCUS08306. PMID: 19335128.

[2] Menon G, Hegde A. Moyamoya disease. Arch Med Health Sci. 2019;7(2): 224-232

[3] Suzuki J, Takaku A. Cerebrovascular "moyamoya" disease. Disease showing abnormal net-like vessels in base of brain. Arch Neurol. 1969 Mar;20(3):288-99. doi: 10.1001/archneur.1969.00480090076012. PMID: 5775283.

[4] Phi JH, Wang KC, Lee JY, Kim SK. Moyamoya Syndrome: A Window of Moyamoya Disease. J Korean Neurosurg Soc. 2015 Jun;57(6):408-14. doi: 10.3340/jkns.2015.57.6.408. Epub 2015 Jun 30. PMID: 26180607; PMCID: PMC4502236.

[5] Research Committee on the Pathology and Treatment of Spontaneous Occlusion of the Circle of Willis; Health Labour Sciences Research Grant for Research on Measures for Intractable Diseases. Guidelines for diagnosis and treatment of moyamoya disease (spontaneous occlusion of the circle of Willis). Neurol Med Chir (Tokyo). 2012;52(5):245-66. doi: 10.2176/nmc.52.245. PMID: 22870528.

[6] Kim JS. Moyamoya Disease: Epidemiology, Clinical Features, and Diagnosis. J Stroke. 2016 Jan;18(1):2-11. doi: 10.5853/jos.2015.01627. Epub 2016 Jan 29. PMID: 26846755; PMCID: PMC4747069.

[7] Kamada F, Aoki Y, Narisawa A, Abe Y, Komatsuzaki S, Kikuchi A, Kanno J, Niihori T, Ono M, Ishii N, Owada Y, Fujimura M, Mashimo Y, Suzuki Y, Hata A, Tsuchiya S, Tominaga T, Matsubara Y, Kure S. A genome-wide association study identifies RNF213 as the first Moyamoya disease gene. J Hum Genet. 2011 Jan;56(1):34-40. doi: 10.1038/jhg.2010.132. Epub 2010 Nov 4. PMID: 21048783.

[8] Baba T, Houkin K, Kuroda S. Novel epidemiological features of moyamoya disease. J Neurol Neurosurg Psychiatry. 2008 Aug;79(8):900-4. doi: 10.1136/jnnp.2007.130666. Epub 2007 Dec 12. PMID: 18077479.

[9] Uchino K, Johnston SC, Becker KJ, Tirschwell DL. Moyamoya disease in Washington State and California. Neurology. 2005 Sep 27;65(6):956-8. doi: 10.1212/01.wnl.0000176066.33797.82. PMID: 16186547

[10] Wakai K, Tamakoshi A, Ikezaki K, Fukui M, Kawamura T, Aoki R, et al. Epidemiological features of Moyamoya disease in Japan: findings from a nationwide survey. Clinical Neurology and Neurosurgery. 1997 Oct; 99:S1-5.

[11] Chen Pei-Chun, Yang Shih-Hung, Chien Kuo-Liong, Tsai I-Ju, Kuo Meng-Fai. Epidemiology of Moyamoya Disease in Taiwan. Stroke. 2014 May 1;45(5):1258-63

[12] Ahn IM, Park DH, Hann HJ, Kim KH, Kim HJ, Ahn HS. Incidence, prevalence, and survival of moyamoya disease in Korea: a nationwide, population-based study. Stroke. 2014 Apr;45(4):1090-5. doi: 10.1161/STROKEAHA.113.004273. Epub 2014 Mar 4. PMID: 24595588.

[13] Zhang H, Zheng L, Feng L. Epidemiology, diagnosis and treatment of moyamoya disease. Exp Ther Med. 2019 Mar;17(3):1977-1984. doi: 10.3892/etm.2019.7198. Epub 2019 Jan 25. PMID: 30867689; PMCID: PMC6395994.

[14] Sun SJ, Zhang JJ, Li ZW, Xiong ZW, Wu XL, Wang S, Shu K, Chen JC. Histopathological features of middle cerebral artery and superficial temporal artery from patients with moyamoya disease and enlightenments on clinical treatment. J Huazhong Univ Sci Technolog Med Sci. 2016 Dec;36(6):871-875. doi: 10.1007/s11596-016-1677-5. Epub 2016 Dec 7. PMID: 27924520.

[15] Masuda J, Ogata J, Yutani C. Smooth muscle cell proliferation and localization of macrophages and T cells in the occlusive intracranial major arteries in moyamoya disease. Stroke. 1993 Dec;24(12):1960-7. doi: 10.1161/01.str.24.12.1960. PMID: 7902623

[16] Oka K, Yamashita M, Sadoshima S, Tanaka K. Cerebral haemorrhage in Moyamoya disease at autopsy. Virchows Arch A Pathol Anat Histol. 1981;392(3):247-61. doi: 10.1007/BF02155663. PMID: 7269227.

[17] Kono S, Oka K, Sueishi K. Histopathologic and morphometric studies of leptomeningeal vessels in moyamoya disease. Stroke. 1990 Jul;21(7):1044-50. doi: 10.1161/01.str.21.7.1044. PMID: 2368105.

[18] Ikeda H, Sasaki T, Yoshimoto T, Fukui M, Arinami T. Mapping of a familial moyamoya disease gene to chromosome 3p24.2-p26. *Am J Hum Genet*. 1999;64(2):533-537. doi:10.1086/302243

[19] Guey S, Tournier-Lasserve E, Hervé D, Kossorotoff M. Moyamoya disease and syndromes: from genetics to clinical management. Appl Clin Genet. 2015 Feb 16;8:49-68. doi: 10.2147/TACG.S42772. PMID: 25733922; PMCID: PMC4337618.

[20] Tanigawara T, Yamada H, Sakai N, Andoh T, Deguchi K, Iwamura M. Studies on cytomegalovirus and Epstein-Barr virus infection in moyamoya disease. Clin Neurol Neurosurg. 1997 Oct;99 Suppl 2:S225-8. doi: 10.1016/s0303-8467(97)00049-8. PMID: 9409443.

[21] Gupta A, Tyagi A, Romo M, Amoroso KC, Sonia F. Moyamoya Disease: A Review of Current Literature. *Cureus*. 2020;12(8):e10141. Published 2020 Aug 30. doi:10.7759/cureus.10141

[22] Fernandez-Alvarez E, Pineda M, Royo C, Manzanares R. "Moya-moya" disease caused by cranial trauma. Brain Dev. 1979;1(2):133-8. doi: 10.1016/s0387-7604(79)80022-4. PMID: 121867.

[23] Bitzer M, Topka H. Progressive cerebral occlusive disease after radiation therapy. Stroke. 1995 Jan;26(1):131-6. doi: 10.1161/01.str.26.1.131. PMID: 7839383.

[24] Kuriyama S, Kusaka Y, Fujimura M, Wakai K, Tamakoshi A, Hashimoto S, Tsuji I, Inaba Y, Yoshimoto T. Prevalence and clinicoepidemiological features of moyamoya disease in Japan: findings from a nationwide epidemiological survey. Stroke. 2008 Jan;39(1):42-7. doi: 10.1161/STROKEAHA.107.490714. Epub 2007 Nov 29. PMID: 18048855.

[25] Zipfel GJ, Fox DJ Jr, Rivet DJ. Moyamoya disease in adults: the role of cerebral revascularization. *Skull Base*. 2005;15(1):27-41. doi:10.1055/s-2005-868161

[26] Scott RM, Smith JL, Robertson RL, Madsen JR, Soriano SG, Rockoff MA. Long-term outcome in children with moyamoya syndrome after cranial revascularization by pial synangiosis. J Neurosurg. 2004 Feb;100(2 Suppl Pediatrics):142-9. doi: 10.3171/ped.2004.100.2.0142. PMID: 14758941.

[27] Seol HJ, Wang KC, Kim SK, Hwang YS, Kim KJ, Cho BK. Headache in pediatric moyamoya disease: review of 204 consecutive cases. J Neurosurg.

2005 Nov;103(5 Suppl):439-42. doi: 10.3171/ped.2005.103.5.0439. PMID: 16302616.

[28] Kim DS, Ko TS, Ra YS, Choi CG. Postoperative electroencephalogram for follow up of pediatric Moyamoya disease. J Korean Med Sci. 2006 Jun;21(3):495-9. doi: 10.3346/jkms.2006.21.3.495. PMID: 16778396; PMCID: PMC2729958.

[29] Smith ER, Scott RM. Moyamoya: epidemiology, presentation, and diagnosis. Neurosurg Clin N Am. 2010 Jul;21(3):543-51. doi: 10.1016/j.nec.2010.03.007. PMID: 20561502.

[30] Mugikura S, Takahashi S, Higano S, Shirane R, Sakurai Y, Yamada S. Predominant involvement of ipsilateral anterior and posterior circulations in moyamoya disease. Stroke. 2002 Jun;33(6):1497-500. doi: 10.1161/01.str.0000016828.62708.21. PMID: 12052981.

[31] Yasaka M, Ogata T, Yasumori K, Inoue T, Okada Y. Bottle neck sign of the proximal portion of the internal carotid artery in moyamoya disease. J Ultrasound Med. 2006 Dec;25(12):1547-52; quiz 1553-4. doi: 10.7863/jum.2006.25.12.1547. PMID: 17121949.

[32] Kodama N, Aoki Y, Hiraga H, Wada T, Suzuki J. Electroencephalographic findings in children with moyamoya disease. Arch Neurol. 1979 Jan;36(1):16-9. doi: 10.1001/archneur.1979.00500370046008. PMID: 420596.

[33] Kim T, Oh CW, Bang JS, Kim JE, Cho WS. Moyamoya Disease: Treatment and Outcomes. *J Stroke*. 2016;18(1): 21-30. doi:10.5853/jos.2015.01739

[34] Kuroda S, Ishikawa T, Houkin K, Nanba R, Hokari M, Iwasaki Y. Incidence and clinical features of disease progression in adult moyamoya disease. Stroke. 2005 Oct;36(10):2148-53. doi: 10.1161/01.STR.0000182256.32489.99. Epub 2005 Sep 22. PMID: 16179571.

[35] Cho WS, Chung YS, Kim JE, Jeon JP, Son YJ, Bang JS, Kang HS, Sohn CH, Oh CW. The natural clinical course of hemodynamically stable adult moyamoya disease. J Neurosurg. 2015 Jan;122(1):82-9. doi: 10.3171/2014.9.JNS132281. PMID: 25361479.

[36] Kuroda S, Shiga T, Ishikawa T, Houkin K, Narita T, Katoh C, Tamaki N, Iwasaki Y. Reduced blood flow and preserved vasoreactivity characterize oxygen hypometabolism due to incomplete infarction in occlusive carotid artery diseases. J Nucl Med. 2004 Jun;45(6):943-9. PMID: 15181128.

[37] Macyszyn L, Attiah M, Ma TS, Ali Z, Faught R, Hossain A, Man K, Patel H, Sobota R, Zager EL, Stein SC. Direct versus indirect revascularization procedures for moyamoya disease: a comparative effectiveness study. J Neurosurg. 2017 May;126(5):1523-1529. doi: 10.3171/2015.8.JNS15504. Epub 2016 Jul 29. PMID: 27471892.

[38] Yamada S, Oki K, Itoh Y, Kuroda S, Houkin K, Tominaga T, Miyamoto S, Hashimoto N, Suzuki N; Research Committee on Spontaneous Occlusion of Circle of Willis (Moyamoya Disease). Effects of Surgery and Antiplatelet Therapy in Ten-Year Follow-Up from the Registry Study of Research Committee on Moyamoya Disease in Japan. J Stroke Cerebrovasc Dis. 2016 Feb;25(2):340-9. doi: 10.1016/j.jstrokecerebrovasdis.2015.10.003. Epub 2015 Nov 30. PMID: 26654669.

[39] Rosi A, Riordan CP, Smith ER, Scott RM, Orbach DB. Clinical status and evolution in moyamoya: which angiographic findings correlate? Brain Commun. 2019 Oct 30;1(1):fcz029. doi: 10.1093/braincomms/fcz029. PMID: 32954269; PMCID: PMC7425301.

[40] Kim T, Oh CW, Kwon OK, Hwang G, Kim JE, Kang HS, Cho WS, Bang JS. Stroke prevention by direct revascularization for patients with adult-onset moyamoya disease presenting with ischemia. J Neurosurg. 2016 Jun;124(6):1788-93. doi: 10.3171/2015.6.JNS151105. Epub 2015 Dec 4. Erratum in: J Neurosurg. 2016 Jun;124(6):1875. PMID: 26636391.

[41] Noh HJ, Kim SJ, Kim JS, Hong SC, Kim KH, Jun P, Bang OY, Chung CS, Lee KH, Lee KH, Kim GM. Long term outcome and predictors of ischemic stroke recurrence in adult moyamoya disease. J Neurol Sci. 2015 Dec 15;359(1-2):381-8. doi: 10.1016/j.jns.2015.11.018. Epub 2015 Nov 10. PMID: 26671146.

[42] Guzman R, Lee M, Achrol A, Bell-Stephens T, Kelly M, Do HM, Marks MP, Steinberg GK. Clinical outcome after 450 revascularization procedures for moyamoya disease. Clinical article. J Neurosurg. 2009 Nov;111(5):927-35. doi: 10.3171/2009.4.JNS081649. PMID: 19463046.

Section 3

Clinical Features of Moyamoya Disease

Chapter 3

Clinical Aspects of Moyamoya Disease

Sandhya Manorenj and Reshma Sultana Shaik

Abstract

Moyamoya disease is a chronic progressive, non-atherosclerotic, occlusive intracranial vasculopathy involving major cerebral arteries around the circle of Willis. MMD occurs frequently in East Asian populations but the disease can affect the American and European ethnicities as well. Knowledge of clinical aspects of Moyamoya disease (MMD) is important in view of distinctive clinical presentation observed in children and adults. MMD has bimodal age of distribution, with peaks in the first and last decades of life. Childhood MMD is characterised by Ischemic manifestation (Transient ischemic attack, Cerebral Infarction), whereas adult MMD presents with hemorrhagic manifestations (Intracerebral haemorrhage, Intraventricular bleed). Refractory headache, seizure and ophthalmological abnormalities are other clinical presentations of MMD. A high index of clinical suspicion and an eye to recognise the common as well as unusual manifestations of the disease and inciting events may prevent delay in the diagnosis. A thorough knowledge about the varied clinical presentation would aid clinician for early diagnosis and management of this rare entity. The present article provides extensive review on the clinical aspects of MMD amongst adults and paediatric population, on the basis of previous articles and research studies.

Keywords: Moyamoya disease, Moyamoya syndrome, clinical features

1. Introduction

Takeuchi and Shimizu Takeuchi first described Moyamoya disease, in 1957 [1]. The term "Moyamoya" was coined to this illness due to its angiographic appearance of "something hazy, like a puff of cigarette smoke" (Moyamoya in Japanese) [1] "Moyamoya disease" (MMD) and "Moyamoya syndrome" (MMS) are both chronic cerebrovascular diseases affecting distal internal carotid and proximal portions of the anterior and middle cerebral arteries [2]. Though Moyamoya disease and Moyamoya syndrome are used synonymously, a subtle distinction separates these two entities. Moyamoya vasculopathy in those with underlying risk factors are described under the umbrella term "Moyamoya syndrome", thus a wide variety of conditions can incite a Moyamoya vasculopathy, however, if a similar angiographic appearance is evident in those with no risk factors, except for an underlying genetic predisposition, it is entitled as "Moyamoya disease" [2]. One more distinction is the" bilateral "angiographic appearance pathognomonic for Moyamoya disease, whilst" unilateral "vasculopathy always qualifies to a Moyamoya syndrome, even without an underlying associated risk factor [2].

2. Literature research strategy

We searched PubMed from 1968 to January 2021 with the words "Moyamoya disease", "Moyamoya syndrome", "population-based", "epidemiology", "risk factors", "genetics", "clinical aspects",clinical features of Moyamoya, seizure and Moyamoya, headache and Moyamoya, paediatric Moyamoya, Adult Moyamoya, stroke and Moyamoya, neuropsychological profile of Moyamoya, Research studies on Moyamoya, Case reports of Moyamoya. Relevant articles were also searched in the national and International journals where the full article could be retrieved. Clinical manifestation and underlying pathophysiology was reviewed in the searched article to provide an extensive review ofclinical aspects of Moyamoya disease.

2.1 Epidemiology

This disease entity was believed to affect Asian heritage, given their genetic predisposition. However, it is now a well-known fact that this disease entity can affect American and European ethnicities [3]. This disease has a bimodal distribution of age-specific incidence rates with two peaks in the age groups of 5 years in children andmid-40s in the adults [3, 4]. It is twice more common in females as in males [3]. The incidence estimates of 0.35–0.54/100,000 are found in the Japanese and Korean populations [5]. An incidence of 0.086 cases per 100,000 persons inAmericans, incidence-rate ratios are 4.6 for Asian Americans, 2.2 for blacks, and 0.5 for Hispanics [6].

2.2 Etiopathogenesis

Moyamoya disease has a genetic aetiology, as mentioned above. Many studies where total genome search linkage was performed found an association between the disease and markers located at 3p24.2–26 chromosome [7], a possible connection of the marker D6S441 located on chromosome 6 which also has HLA gene [8], linkage to chromosome 17 have also been reported.

Moyamoya syndrome is associated with many conditions, as described below: [8].

Chromosomal/Genetic disorder	**Neurofibromatosis, "Down's syndrome, Turner syndrome**
Haematological disorders	Sickle cell anaemia, Thalassemia, Aplastic anaemia
Infectious disease	Leptospirosis, Tuberculous meningitis
Neoplasms	Craniopharyngioma, Wilms tumour
Drug abuse	Phenobarbital
Autoimmune diseases	"Behcet's disease, "Sjögren's syndrome, systemic lupus erythematosus (SLE), Henoch Scholein Purpura (HSP) and 'Graves' disease
Others	Cardiomyopathy, Polycystic kidney, Pulmonary sarcoidosis, Irradiation, Trauma, Renal artery stenosis

A role of fibroblast growth factor, prostaglandin, and activation of cox2 in the vascular smooth muscle, EBV DNA and propionibacteria have all been proposed as a possible mediator of the neovascular response [9].

2.3 Natural history

Disease progression can be slow, with overlapping intermittent events, or it can be a fulminant course, with rapid neurologic decline [10]. It has been reported that symptomatic progression is observed for five years, and delay in the rap initiation may have catastrophic consequences [10].

3. Diagnostic criteria

Various guidelines have been published over time and again. In 1996 and 1997 Japan published diagnostic criteria for the pathology and treatment of MMD [11]. In 2012, Japan published the latest guidelines based on 1997 guidelines [11].

Though cerebral angiography remains the gold standard for the diagnosis (**Table 1**), novel guidelines added a staging based on scores of magnetic resonance (MR) angiography (MRA) [12].

Stenosis or occlusion at the end of ICA and/or the initial segment of the ACA and/or MCA.

At least two obvious shadows of the blood flow are displayed on the same scan level at the basal ganglia region, suggesting the existence of an abnormal vascular network.

The above manifestations are bilateral, but bilateral lesions may be staged differently.

The total score was the sum total of MRA results and each side (right and left were scored individually) as shown in the **Tables 2** and **3**.

As per the new guidelines, other diseases viz. atherosclerosis, autoimmune diseases, meningitis, brain tumours, Down syndrome, Recklinghausen's disease, head injury and cerebrovascular damage after head irradiation, should be excluded [12].

Pathological findings suggestive of MMD are fibrocellular thickening of arterial intima, waviness of internal elastic lamina, thinning of the media, variable stenosis and occlusion of the implicated vessels, presence of anastomotic and perforating branches around the circle of Willis and pial reticular conglomerate of small blood vessels [12].

Definitive MMD: Either angiographic or MRA appearance of vessels bilaterally with the exclusion of alternative diagnosis [13].

Stage	Cerebral angiographic findings
I	Narrowing of the carotid fork
II	Initiation of the moyamoya (dilated major cerebral artery and a slight moyamoya vessel network)
III	Intensification of the moyamoya (disappearance of the middle and anterior cerebral arteries, and thick and distinct moyamoya vessels)
IV	Minimization of the moyamoya (disappearance of the posterior cerebral artery, and narrowing of individual moyamoya vessels)
V	Reduction of the moyamoya (disappearance of all the main cerebral arteries arising from the internal carotid artery system, further minimization of the moyamoya vessels, and an increase in the collateral pathways from the external carotid artery system)
VI	Disappearance of the moyamoya (disappearance of the moyamoya vessels, with cerebral blood flow derived only from the external carotid artery and the vertebrobasilar artery systems)

Table 1.
Stages and cerebral angiographic findings.

Scoring for each artery	
Score	**MRA Findings**
Internal carotid artery	
0	Normal
1	Stenosis of C1
2	Discontinuity of the C1 signal
3	Invisible
Middle cerebral artery	
0	Normal
1	Stenosis of M1
2	Discontinuity of the M1 signal
3	Invisible
Anterior cerebral artery	
0	Normal A2 and blood vessels distal to A2
1	Signal decrease A2 and its distal blood vessels
2	Invisible
Posterior cerebral artery	
0	Normal P2 and blood vessels distal to P2
1	Signal decrease P2 and its distal blood vessels
2	Invisible

Table 2.
Classification and scoring based on the MRA findings.

MRA total score	MRA stage
0–1	1
2–4	2
5–7	3
8–10	4

Table 3.
Total score calculated individually for the right and left side.

Probable MMD: Either angiographic or MRA appearance of vessels unilaterally with the exclusion of alternative diagnosis [13]. Unilateral MMD may progress to bilateral MMD in 10 to 39% of the cases.

If the autopsy is performed with no previous angiography, pathological findings similar to those mentioned above may serve in the diagnosis of MMD [13].

Quasi MMD or Rui MMD:Evidence of stenosis or occlusion of distal ICA or proximal MCA or ACA with abnormal vascular network either unilateral or bilateral, in association with an underlying disease [13]. Concurrent occurrence of congenital disease is common in children, and acquired disorderis common in adults.

Unstable MMD: Defined as "rapid progression or repeated stroke". It is a clinically challenging condition. It is more prevalent in patients younger than threeyears and those with an associated underlying disease. It is a possible risk factor associated with perioperative ischemic complication [14].

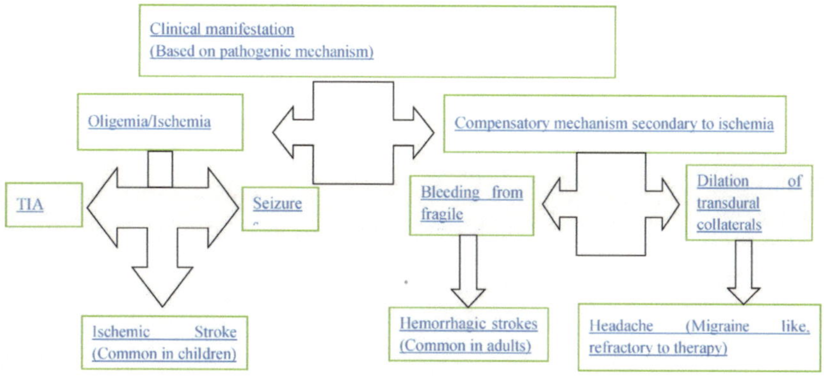

Figure 1.
Flow chart showing the clinical manifestation of Moyamoya disease based on underlying pathogenic mechanism.

Moyamoya disease/syndrome symptoms can be broadly categorised into two, by the underlying mechanism (**Figure 1**). The first category of symptoms is oligemia like transient ischemic attack (TIA), stroke, and oligemia like transient ischemic attack (TIA), stroke, and seizures. Amongst the ischemic symptoms, completed strokes are more common in children, a possible explanation being their inability to identify and complain about TIAs [11]. The second category of symptoms are due to the compensatory mechanisms' harmful consequences to ischemia like a haemorrhage from fragile collateral vessels and headaches from dilated transdural collaterals [10].

"Initial attacks" of MMD [12].

The research committee has identified nine types of initial episodes of MMD.

Hemorrhagic type.

Epileptic type.

Infarction type (can be same side or alternating hemiplegia).

TIA type.

Frequent TIA type (two or more attacks per month).

Headache type.

Asymptomatic type.

Other types.

Details unknown type.

4. Clinical manifestations in children

Moyamoya disease presents with ischemic symptoms in children, an incidence of 68% and adults usually present with a hemorrhagic stroke, about 42% [10].

Amongst the ischemic symptoms, completed strokes are more common in children, a possible explanation being their inability to identify and complain about TIAs [15]. They can be transient or fixed. Most commonly occur in the territory of the internal carotid artery and proximal middle and anterior cerebral arteries [10].

Underlying mechanism:

Progressive stenosis of the internal carotid and middle cerebral arteries are responsible for most of the symptoms [10].

Maximally dilated cortical vessels in patients with chronic ischemia, constrict in response to the decreased carbon dioxide due to hyperventilation, resulting in reduced cerebral perfusion and thus exacerbating the symptoms [16].

Precipitating factors: [16].

Crying (In the paediatric population).
Hyperventilation (In paediatric population).
Exercise.
Anaesthesia.
Dehydration.
Altitude.
Eating a hot meal.
Focal Symptoms: [10].
Hemiparesis.
Dysarthria.
Aphasia.
Visual deficits.
Chorea.
Non-focal symptoms: [10].

Headache: Approximately 20% of the paediatric patients under the age of 14 years suffer from headache. Likely explananation for the headache was the reduction of cerebral blood flow or cerebral blood flow reserve and diffusive cortical inhibition [17]. Dilatation of meningeal and leptomeningeal collateral vessels may stimulate dural nociceptors. Every refractory headache, especially in the paediatric population should be thoroughly worked up for moyamoya disease [17] Headaches can be migraine-like episodes which may respond to revascularization surgery or remain refractory to surgery [17].

Cognitive impairment, learning disability, and attention deficits.
Seizures.
Syncope.

Personality change, mistaken for a psychiatric illness like schizophrenia, acute transient psychosis, and mania [18].

Symptoms and signs which serve as biomarkers in MMD/MMS:

Orthostatic intolerance (also termed "orthostatic dysregulation"): [19] Orthostatic intolerance is defined as" a disturbance in the physiological adjustment mechanism compensating for physical stresses, such as standing, and causes a variety of symptoms associated with hemodynamic or autonomic nervous system compromise". These symptoms can have a potential impact on the quality of life of paediatric MMD patients. In a study done by H. Uchino et al., 59% of children 10–15 years old suffered from orthostatic intolerance. These symptoms usually go unnoticed, and thus a thorough history from the patients and their caretakers become mandatory.

Symptoms which are suggestive of orthostatic intolerance:
Frequent headache.
Susceptibility to vertigo & dizziness on standing.
Fatigue.
Difficulty while getting out of bed.
Motion sickness.
Palpitation &/or dyspnea after mild exercise.
Tendency for fainting in the standing position.
Anorexia.
Occasional umbilical colic (severe abdominal pain).
Nausea on taking a hot bath or encountering unpleasant experiences.
Absent from school due to the above symptoms.
Pallor.

Fundus: Retinovascular anomalies and "morning glory disk" an enlargement of the optic disk should compel the clinician to look for moyamoya vasculopathy [20]. Morning glory syndrome or Morning glory disc anomaly is an unusual

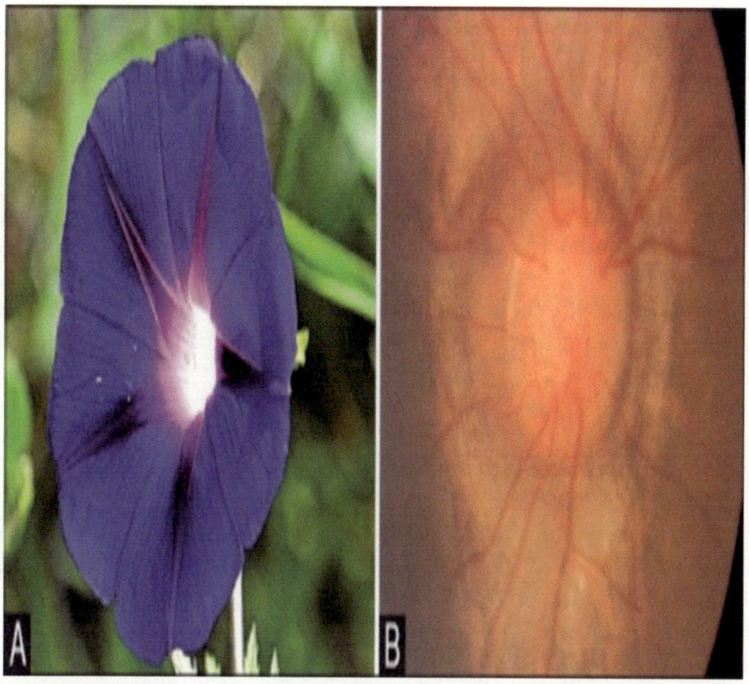

Figure 2.
*Showing morning glory disc [courtesy:Indian J Radiol imaging. 2018 Apr-Jun] [22]. MRI brain CISS sequence of orbit region may further confirm funnel-shaped excavation of the posterior globein morning glory syndrome of Moyamoya disease (**Figure 3**) [22].*

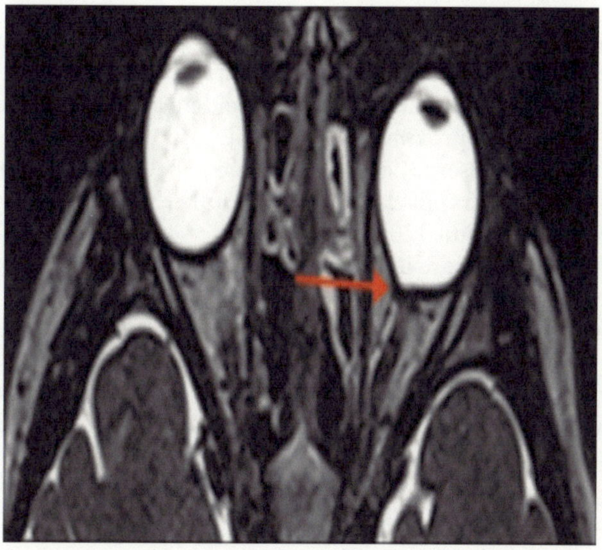

Figure 3.
Showing funnel-shaped excavation of posterior globe [courtesy: Indian J Radiol imaging. 2018 Apr-Jun] [22].

congenital optic disc anomaly characterised by a funnel-shaped excavation of the posterior globe that incorporates the optic disc [21]. Kindler described it in 1970 because it resembled the morning glory flower. The disc itself is enlarged, and orange or pink in colour within a surrounding area of peripapillary chorioretinal pigmentary changes. Alteration of lamina cribrosa and posterior sclera due to embryonic developmental defect leads to this fundus's flowery appearanace.

Presence of this sign indicates an association with systemic or intracranial vasculopathies such as MMD. Morning glory disc occurs in 50% of patients with the MMD (**Figure 2**).

Sequelae of MMD: [16].

Refractory headaches.

Recurrent TIAs.

Posterior cerebral artery (PCA) involvement.

Recurrent intracranial aneurysms.

Unstable MMD.

In children with MMD, recurrent ischemias can result in cerebral atrophy and thus emanate the onset of learning difficulties, cognitive impairment and mental retardation.

5. Clinical manifestations in adults

Hemorrhagic manifestations are more common in adults than in children. These haemorrhages are seen in 42% of the adults. The location of the bleeding can be intraventricular, intraparenchymal or subarachnoid.

Underlying mechanism:

Rupture of fragile collateral vessels as a result of chronic oligemia [23].

Development of cerebral aneurysms at the apex of the basilar artery and posterior communicating artery, areas of increased shear stress due to shifting circulatory pattern at the base of the brain is another source of haemorrhage [24].

Quasi MMD is common in adults, and the manifestations may range from asymptomatic to catastrophic haemorrhage and rebleeding with a moribund prognosis [13].

Ischemic symptoms are more common in the paediatric population, as described above. Amongst the ischemic symptoms transient ischemic attacks(TIA) are more common in the paediatric population with an incidence of 81% and infarctions are experienced by adults in approximately 51% [25].

Reason for the above observation could be due to better development of leptomeningeal collaterals (LMCs) in children than adults [25]. Various factors have been implicated in this observation: [25].

Ageing: Significant decrease in LMCs and increased tortuosity and vascular resistance in leptomeningeal vessels.

Concomitant diseases in adult MMD patients like hypertension may have an effect on the development of collaterals.

Focal cerebral ischemia may stimulate cytokines' secretion, such as angiogenic peptides and vascular endothelial growth factor (VEGF). These cytokines levels are lower in adults.

Associated underlying conditions are commonly observed in adults with MMD.

Clinical clues for associated disorders: [10].

History of radiotherapy	Head and neck malignancies like optic gliomas, craniopharyngiomas, and pituitary tumours
Endocrine insufficiency	Neurofibromas or tumours compressing hypothalamic–optic pathway and pituitary stalk
Visual field defects	Tumours compressing hypothalamic–optic pathway, Strokes involving the visual pathway
Anaemia	Sickle cell anaemia, Thalassemia, Aplastic anaemia
Acute abdomen, bone crises	Sickle cell anaemia

Neurocutaneous markers	Neurofibromatosis, Down's syndrome,Turner syndrome
Refractory hypertension	Renal Artery Stenosis
Fever	Leptospirosis, CNS tuberculosis
Recurrent falls (Especially in the Paediatric population)	TIAs
Systemic symptoms like cutaneous rash, joint pains	SLE, Sjogren syndrome and HSP

Special Precautions to be exercised:

EEG: Hyperventilation may precipitate an acute oligemic episode, thus caution has been exercised in patients with suspected moyamoya disease. Specific alterations in MMD/MMS have characteristic changes in EEG, consisting of the gradual decrease in frequency and amplitude activation after hyperventilation. These EEG changes are referred to as re-build-up phenomenon [2].

Anaesthesia and postop care.

Travelling to high altitudes.

Exercise.

6. Conclusion

A vast constellation of symptoms constitutes a repertoire in MMD. They may facilitate the diagnosis or add more confusion to the diagnosis. Fundus examination and characteristic angiogram findings clinch the diagnosis of MMD. A high index of clinical suspicion and an eye to recognise the disease's common and unusual manifestations and inciting events may prevent delay in the diagnosis. Early recognition of illness with prompt treatment may halt the progression and allay catastrophic neurological deficits.

Author details

Sandhya Manorenj* and Reshma Sultana Shaik
Princess Esra Hospital, Deccan College of Medical Sciences, Hyderabad, India

*Address all correspondence to: drsandhyamanorenj@gmail.com

References

[1] Takeuchi K SK. Hypogenesis of bilateral internal carotid arteries. No To Shinkei. 1957;9: 37-43.

[2] Scott RM, Smith ER. Moyamoya Disease and Moyamoya Syndrome. N Engl J Med. 2009;360(12):1226-37.

[3] Wakai K, Tamakoshi A, Ikezaki K E al. Epidemiological features of moyamoya disease in Japan: findings from a nationwide survey. Clin Neurol Neurosurg. 1997;99(Suppl 2):S1-5.

[4] Suzuki J KN. Moyamoya disease — a review. Stroke. 1983;14:104-9.

[5] Kuriyama S, Kusaka Y, Fujimura M, Wakai K TA, Hashimoto S et al. Prevalence and clinicoepidemiological features of moyamoya disease in Japan: Findingsfrom a nationwide epidemiological survey. Stroke. 2008;(39):42-7.

[6] Uchino K, Johnston SC BK, DL. T. Moyamoya disease in Washington State and California. Neurology. 2005;(65):956-8.

[7] Ikeda H, Sasaki T YT et al. Mapping of a familial moyamoya disease gene to chromosome 3p24.2-p.26. Am J Hum Genet. 1999;64:533-7.

[8] Inoue TK, lkezaki K ST et al. Linkage analysis of moyamoya disease on chromosome 6. J Child Neurol. 2000;(15):179-82.

[9] Gosalakkal JA. Moyamoya disease: A review. Neurol India. 2002;50(1):6-10.

[10] Scott RM, Smith JL RR, Madsen JR, Soriano SG RM. Long-term outcome in children with moyamoya syndrome after cranial revascularization by pial synangiosis. J Neurosurg. 2004;(100):142-9.

[11] TNCoHS C and C, PatoissecoS. Chinese expert consensus on diagnosis and treatment of moyamoya disease and moyamoya syndrome. Chin J Neurosurg. 2017;(6):541-7.

[12] Research Committee on the Pathology and Treatment of Spontaneous Occlusion of the Circle of Willis; Health Labour Sciences Research Grant for Research on Measures for Intractable Diseases: Guidelines for diagnosis and treatment of moyamoya disease. Neurol Med Chir. 2012;(52):245-66.

[13] Guidelines for Diagnosis and Treatment of Moyamoya Disease (Spontaneous Occlusion of the Circle of Willis). In: Neurologia medico-chirurgica. 2012. p. 245-66.

[14] Funaki T, Takahashi JC, Takagi Y, Kikuchi T, Yoshida K, Mitsuhara T, et al. Unstable moyamoya disease: Clinical features and impact on perioperative ischemic complications. J Neurosurg. 2015;122(2):400-7.

[15] Jea A, Smith ER, Robertson R S, RM. Moyamoya syndrome associated with Down syndrome: outcome after surgical revascularization. Pediatrics. 2005;116(5):e694-701.

[16] Tagawa T, Naritomi H MT, Yabuuchi H ST. Regional cerebral blood flow, clinical manifestations, and age in children with moyamoya disease. Stroke. 1987;18:906-10.

[17] Seol HJ, Wang KC, Kim SK, Hwang YS KK and CB. Headache in pediatric moyamoya disease: Review of 204 consecutive cases. J Neurosurg. 2005;103(5):S439-42.

[18] Lubman DI, Pantelis C DP, Proffitt TM VD. Moyamoya disease in a patient with schizophrenia. J Int Neuropsychol Soc. 2003;9:806-10.

[19] Uchino H, Kazumata K, Ito M, Nakayama N, Houkin K. Novel insights into symptomatology of moyamoya disease in pediatric patients: Survey of symptoms suggestive of orthostatic intolerance. J Neurosurg Pediatr. 2017;20(5):485-8.

[20] Massaro M, Thorarensen O LG, Maguire AM, Zimmerman RA B, MC. Morning glory disc anomaly and moyamoya vessels. Arch Ophthalmol. 1998;(116):253-4.

[21] Quah BL, Hamilton J, Blaser S, Héon E TN. Morning glory disc anomaly, midline cranial defects and abnormal carotid circulation: An association worth looking for. Pediatr Radiol. 2005;(35):525-8.

[22] J P. Morning glory syndrome with Moyamoya disease: A rare association with role of imaging. Indian J Radiol Imaging. 2018;28(2):165-8.

[23] Iwama T, Morimoto M HN, Goto Y, Todaka T SM. Mechanism of intracranial rebleeding in moyamoya disease. Clin Neurol Neurosurg. 1997;99(2):S187-90.

[24] Kawaguchi S, Sakaki T MT, Kakizaki T KK. Characteristics of intracranial aneurysms associated with moyamoya disease: a review of 111 cases. Acta Neurochir. 1996;138:1287-94.

[25] Liu ZW, Han C, Wang H, Zhang Q, Li SJ, Bao X yang, et al. Clinical characteristics and leptomeningeal collateral status in pediatric and adult patients with ischemic moyamoya disease. CNS Neurosci Ther. 2020;26(1):14-20.

Section 4

Neuropsychological Features of Moyamoya Patients

Chapter 4

Neuropsychology of Moyamoya Disease

Raúl Espert and Marien Gadea

Abstract

Moyamoya disease (MMD) is an occlusive cerebrovascular disease characterized by progressive stenosis or occlusion in the terminal portion of the bilateral internal carotid arteries, and affect both children and adults. In this pathology, which presents itself through ischemia or cerebral hemorrhage, an unusual compensatory vascular network (moyamoya vessels) develops at the brain's base in the form of collateral channels. MMD can present clinically as hemiparesis, dysarthria, aphasia, headache, seizures, visual deficits, syncope, or personality changes. Neuropsychologically, and even in the absence of obvious stroke, patients often present impaired attention, memory, behavior, and executive functions. This book chapter reviews the current literature regarding the neuropsychological deficits of MMD both in children and adults.

Keywords: Moyamoya disease, neuropsychology, cognitive outcome, pediatric moyamoya

1. Introduction

Moyamoya disease (MMD) is a rare vascular syndrome most commonly found among the Japanese and other Asiatic peoples, its is chareacterized by the angiographic appearance of widespread cerebral collaterals due to occlusion of one or both internal carotid arteries [1]. The aetiology is unclear, but is perhaps related to an acquired lesion of the blood vessels at the brain's base. MMD was first described in Japan in 1957 by Takeuchi and Shimizu [2]. Although it is more common in Japan, clinical cases of the pathology have been reported in other parts of the world [3]. The incidence of MMD peaks in two age groups: int those around 4 years-old (pediatric MoyaMoya Disease, pMMD), and those in their 40s (adult MoyaMoya Disease, aMMD) [4]. There are almost twice as many female patients as there are male [5]. MMD is the most common pediatric cerebrovascular disorder in Japan, with a prevalence of about three cases per 100,000 children [6], while the incidence in Europe is approximately one- tenth of that observed in Japan [7]. A 2005 review result suggest an incidence of 0.086 cases per 100,000 people in the U.S. [8]. There are two main etiological categories of symptoms: those due to cerebral ischemia (stroke, transient ischemic attacks, and seizures, more frequent in pMMD) [9], and hemorrhagic symptoms due to the secondary effects of compensatory mechanisms that are triggered in response to the ischemia (hemorrhage of fragile collateral vessels and headache due to dilated transdural vessels, more frequent in aMMD). Individual variations in the degree of arterial involvement, the progression of stenosis, the regions of the ischemic cortex, and the response to reduced blood supply explain the wide range of clinical presentations of the disease [10]. This chapter reviews the literature on moyamoya disease, specifically on neuropsychological aspects, in both pediatric and adult populations.

2. Pediatric Moyamoya disease (pMMD)

During the onset of Pediatric Moyamoya disease (pMMD), progressive occlusion occurs at the end of the intracranial internal carotid artery, and compensatory net-like abnormal vessels develop in the skull base, generating several clinical symptoms. These collateral vessels mimic a "puff of smoke" when revealed by and angiogram [11]. pMMD can affect both children and adults, but pediatric patients exhibit distinct clinical features, and treatment and prognosies differ from those in adult patients [12].

The distinctive clinical profile of pMMD includes headache, cognitive impairment, hypertension, temporary or permanent blindness, hemiplegia, general paresis of the insane, loss of sensation, aphasia, and mechanisms related to ischemia in the frontal, parietal, and temporal lobes [13, 14]. Children are at a higher risk of suffering Moyamoya Disease (MMD) and the condition is more severe in young children, especially those under four years, in whom the prognosis is often poor [15]. In children, the disease mainly manifests as ischemia, while bleeding is the primary symptom in adults [16]. Despite normal general intellectual functioning, some children with moyamoya disease exhibit cognitive deterioration, primarily learning disability, attention deficit, episodic memory, slow processing speed and neurological abnormalities [17]. Cognitive impairment is not generalized in all children, since some show neuropsychological alterations and others do not. The worst prognosis tends to be seen in children who have had a stroke or cerebral infarction. In contrast, Transient Ischemic Attack (TIA) usually has a better cognitive prognosis [18, 19], with only 15% of patients exhibiting single-domain impairment and 23% showing multiple cognitive domains to be affected after a TIA [20]. The affected area usually includes the terminal portions of the Internal Carotid Arteries (ICAs) and the proximal areas of the anterior or middle cerebral arteries, although Posterior Cerebral Arteries (PCAs) can be affected in some cases [21]. The pattern of cognitive dysfunction is often associated with lesions in frontotemporal areas, with young age [22] and young onset of the disease [23] proving to be the main risk factors for poor neuropsychological outcomes.

Moyamoya disease is characterized by progressive cerebrovascular stenosis with recurrent cerebral ischemic events. TIA attacks are often associated with hyperventilation in children with moyamoya, pointing to hypoperfusion rather than thrombotic vaso-occlusion as a prominent mechanism. The patterns of ischemia and severity of steno-occlusive disease in such children may hold clues to these mechanisms. In this sense, Rafay et al. studied twenty children (between 1 month to 18 years) with MMD in a neuroradiological MRI and angiography [24]. The initial clinical presentation revealed neurological deficits in 17, recurrent TIA in 7, headache in 8, seizures in 8, and alteration in consciousness in 4 children. Infarcts were bilateral in 13 (65%) children (ischemia alone was observed in 14, ischemic stroke with hemorrhagic transformation in two, and primary hemorrhage in two). Infarcts were cortical and/or subcortical in 13 (65%), both deep and cortical watershed in 11 (55%), and cortical watershed alone in 5 (25%) children. The predominant vascular territory involved was the middle cerebral artery. The internal carotid arterial system was involved in all cases, with stage IV being the most frequent angiographic stage. The authors concluded that ischemic injury in deep watershed zones is common in pMMD and may reflect non–vaso-occlusive ischemic mechanisms. They also concluded that the location and severity of the vascular involvement might correlate with various ischemic infarction patterns in MMD and require further study.

In pMMD, a state of chronic ischemia persists in the developing brain, and the possibility of persistent neurologic events and progressive intellectual impairment has been recognized, with no significant correlation detected between age at onset and intellectual quotient (I.Q.) when patients have been monitored from childhood into adulthood [25]. I.Q. begins to decrease after the onset of pMMD, and often stabilizes ten years later [26]. Some studies have reported that 10–30% of patients experience difficulties in school life due to intellectual impairment [27–29]. An analysis of 410 consecutive cases revealed that the overall clinical outcome was excellent in 66%, good in 15%, fair in 15%, and poor in 4% of the patients. According to these results, 81% of the patients had a favorable clinical outcome (excellent or good). Multivariate analyses revealed that infarction on presentation was associated with an unfavorable clinical outcome and decreased vascular reserve only on single-photon emission computerized tomography, with favorable clinical outcome. These results indicate that an early diagnosis and active intervention before irreversible hemodynamic changes take place are essential to achieve a favorable clinical outcome in children with MMD [30]. In 2016 Titsworth, Scott and Smith published a U.S.A. national analysis of 2454 pMMD admissions and the effect of hospital volume on stroke outcome. They concluded that high-volume centres provide significantly improved care and reduced mortality in pediatric moyamoya patients, with the most substantial benefit observed in admissions for surgical revascularization [31].

Tho-Calvi et al. described the characteristics and clinical course of a large UK cohort (eighty-eight) of children with moyamoya attended in multiple centres. When they examined prognostic predictors they concluded that pMMD is associated with multiple recurrences, progressive arteriopathy, and poor outcome in half of patients, especially those who present with arterial ischemic stroke (AIS) and posterior circulation involvement [32]. Cooper et al. evaluated the relationship between neurologic outcome one month after diagnosis of pediatric AIS and motor and adaptive behaviour outcomes at 12 months. Their prospective longitudinal observational cohort study recruited sixty-four children (27 neonates, 19 preschool, and 18 school-aged) from a single children's tertiary hospital who were diagnosed with first AIS between December 2007 and November 2013. Neurologic impairment was evaluated at four time points following AIS diagnosis (at 0 months and 1, 6, and 12 months) using the Pediatric Stroke Outcome Measure (PSOM) or the Recovery and Recurrence Questionnaire. Motor function and adaptive behaviour were assessed at 12 months using standardized measures. Children were grouped for analysis according to age at diagnosis (neonates vs preschool vs school-aged). They concluded that PSOM has value as a predictive tool concerning motor and adaptive behavior when it is used one month after the first AIS has been diagnosed, with variation according to age [33]. In the same line, Funaki, Takahashi and Miyamoto reviewed the long-term outcome of pMMD, focusing on late cerebrovascular events and social outcome of pediatric patients once they reach adulthood. Long-term follow-up data for Asian populations suggested that the incidence of de novo hemorrhage increased at the age of 20 or later, even when 10 years has passed since bypass surgery. According to these authors, social adaptation difficulty, possibly related to cognitive impairment caused by frontal ischemia, continues in 10–20% of patients after they reach adulthood, even though no significant disability is evident in daily life [34].

The pathogenesis of pMMD is unknown. It can result in progressive, irreversible brain function impairment, and an earlier onset corresponds with a worse neuropsychological prognosis. Therefore, evidence-based medical treatment of affected children at an early stage is highly recommended. These treatments consist of direct (intra and extracranial vascular reconstructions, usually involving superficial temporal artery-middle cerebral artery anastomosis) or indirect (multiple burr-hole surgery, encephalomyosynangiosis, and encephaloduroarteriosynangiosis) neurosurgical procedures. This surgery aims to improve the cognitive prognosis, increase the quality of life and reduce the risk of ischemic diseases thanks to improved cerebral hemodynamics [35]. Therefore, compared to adult patients, children with MMD can enjoy a good prognosis if diagnosis and surgical treatment are achieved as soon as possible [36].

In 2018, Kim et al. studied the neuropsychological impacts of indirect revascularization (pre-postoperative) in fifty-five children with MMD. The study was carried out to show that temporal encephaloduroarteriosynangiosis (EDAS) has a positive neuropsychological impact on pMMD patients [37]. The mean age at preoperative evaluation was 9.5 years and the mean age at postoperative evaluation was 10.4. The average interval between initial and follow-up test was ten months. K-WISC-III, the Rey-Kim memory test, the Children's Color Trails Test (CCTT), the Wisconsin Card Sorting Test (WCST), and the Advanced Test of Attention (ATA) were employed to assess patient's neurocognitive profile. Prior to the operation, patients displayed a 54.2% inattention deficit, but only around a 2.5% deficit in verbal memory recall function. After surgery there was a significant increase in performance I.Q. and an improvement of approximately ten scores in memory quotient (M.Q.). The study also reported parietal activation following surgical treatment, which enhanced the ability to interpret visual materials and, which enchanced the ability to interpret visual materials, record, and retrieve visual information. Interestingly, there was a significant improvement in performance in the WCST and CCTT, wich measured prefrontal executive function. Concerning failure to maintain set, no significant postoperative improvements were evident. However, simple and selective visual attention was significantly improved post-operation. The results of neuropsychological field comparison testifies to the effectiveness of temporal EDAS in pediatric MMD patients. This surgical intervention enhances the blood flow in operative areas and improves general cerebral function, including that in frontoparietal domains, leading to an overall improvement in the cognitive function impaired by MMD.

In a sample of thirty children with MMD, Williams et al. [38] examined intellectual and executive functioning. They evaluated the impact of moyamoya type, stroke (clinical or silent), vasculopathy laterality, and disease duration on neurocognitive abilities. All the subjects completed Wechsler Intelligence Scales before therapeutic revascularization procedures were carried out. Reports of executive function were obtained from parents and teachers using the Behavior Rating Index of Executive Function. The children scored significantly lower than the test standardization samples on all indices of intelligence and ratings of executive functioning. The patients did not differ by type of moyamoya or history of stroke. Those with bilateral disease and stroke scored significantly lower than those with unilateral disease on overall intellectual function and verbal comprehension measures. According to teacher ratings, deficits in metacognitive executive functions were even more pronounced in bilateral patients than unilateral ones. Finally, the authors concluded that children with MMD are at risk of intellectual and executive problems, which are exacerbated by bilateral disease and clinical stroke history [38].

Gutierrez-Martignon et al. analyzed the cognitive, academic, and emotional profile of a pediatric case of MMD at diagnosis, on three occasions during evolution (from 9 to 15 years old), before surgery, and after EDAS. An evident cognitive decline in visual attention, processing speed (PS), memory, and visual perception was detected between the first and second evaluations during evolution, while the third evaluation revealed a fluctuating evolution. Executive function, PS, total I.Q., perceptual reasoning, and calculation were most consistently affected during the three assessments, which is consistent with the rest of the literature [39].

The impact on the quality of life of 30 children with MMD (with a median age of 13,5 years) was studied by Ball, Steinberg and Elbers using the Pediatric Quality of Life 4.0 Measurement Model [40]. The authors compared their quality of life to that of chronically ill children and children with stroke in order to better understand the impact of a diagnosis of MMD. The results showed that, even in the absence of stroke, children with moyamoya disease had a lower quality of life than healthy controls and a similar quality of life to chronically ill children and those with non–moyamoya disease stroke. The concluded that hildren with moyamoya disease would benefit from mental health support beyond what a mild physical presentation may indicate.

Assessment of neurological and neuropsychological outcome following revascularization, shows that surgical procedures are effective in halting the neurological progression and results in neuropsychological improvement in some patients [41]. For example, Nehra and Kaur in 2015 reported a male diagnosed with MMD at eight years old and, referred for neuropsychological evaluation at 12 years due to, impaired intellectual functioning with moderate retardation in adaptive social functioning. Two years after psychosocial intervention, the patient showed a remarkable upward trend in his adaptive social functioning and, a jump of 21 I.Q. points in his intellectual functioning [42]. In the same line, Cusin-Lamonica et al. reported the case of a girl of seven years old who suffered two episodes of stroke in the left and right temporal-parietal and left frontal areas that occurred until the age of six years and five months [43]. She presented signs of deterioration in oral and written language (syllabic-alphabetic), non-naming of all graphemes, low arithmetic and writing means, pre-first-grade reading skillsand psycholinguistic delay, and pre-school-level phonological processing skills. The psychological evaluation indicated a satisfactory intellectual level. Revascularization surgery and medication were prescribed.

Considering the infant's brain's developmental plasticity, extrinsic influences, such as psychological interventions for speech-language pathology, coupled with intrinsic influences, can alter the cortical organization and regenerate damaged connections, thus improving the compromised skills of children. A recent systematic review and metaanalysis of pMMD and aMMD, assessed the presence, severity, and nature of cognitive impairments in children and adults with MMD [44]. The authors revised data (collected between 1969 and 2016) pertaining to mean intelligence quotient and standardized z-scores of cognitive tests, and determined percentages of children and adults with cognitive deficits, before and after conservative or surgical treatment. In the case of pMMD, they included 11 studies reporting on a total of 281 children. In children, the median percentage with impaired cognition was 30% (range, 13% to 67%); the median I.Q. was 98 (rang: 71 to 107), and the median z-score was –0.39 for memory, and –0.43 for speed processing. The investigators concluded that many children (30%) with MMD suffer cognitive impairment, with modest to large deficits across various cognitive domains. Thus, extensive prospective studies with a standardized neuropsychological test battery are needed to determine the severity of cognitive impairment and the domains affected.

Recently, Kazumata et al. aimed to investigate cognitive function in the presurgical phase of pediatric patients with MMD with no apparent brain lesions in order to explore an association between cognitive function and cerebral blood flow [45]. They designed a prospective, observational, single-centre study, of 21 children (mean age 10 ± 3.0 years, range 5–14 years) diagnosed with MMD at Hokkaido

University Hospital between 2012 and 2018. A cross-sectional evaluation of intellectual ability was performed using the Wechsler Intelligence Scale for Children. rCBF was measured using [123I] N-isopropyl p-iodoamphetamine/SPECT. The associations among clinical factors, disease severity, regional cerebral blood flow (rCBF), and intelligence test scores were also examined. Results showed that the mean full-scale intelligence quotient (FIQ) was 101.8 ± 12.5 (range 76–125) in children with no apparent brain lesions. A significant difference in the intelligence scale index score was observed most frequently (42.9%) between the working memory index (WMI) and verbal comprehension index. Regional CBF was significantly reduced both in the left and right medial frontal cortices compared to the cerebellum. There was a significant association of rCBF in the left dorsolateral prefrontal cortex (DLPFC) with FIQ, perceptual reasoning index, and processing speed index. Although average intellectual ability was not reduced in the children with MMD, the association of reduced rCBF in the left DLPFC and medial frontal cortex with FIQ, perceptual reasoning and processing speed suggests mild cognitive dysfunction due to cerebral hypoperfusion. Li et al. [46] studied the cognitive performance profile of twenty-one pMMD and its relationship with regional cerebral blood perfusion using arterial spin-labeling magnetic resonance and the Wechsler Intelligence Scale for Children. Results showed that six patients (28.6%) had no cognitive deficits in any index score, while 15 (71.4%) displayed cognitive deficits of varying severity. Nine (42.9%) patients showed overall cognitive impairment, and all cognitive index scores except for Verbal Comprehension Index were significantly lower than the mean scores of normative data than controls of the same age. Perceptual reasoning index was statistically lower in patients with radiologically confirmed cerebral infarction. The area of interest analysis revealed that the left temporal lobe's cerebral blood flow positively correlated with processing speed [46].

The causes of Moyamoya vasculopathy are still unknown, though it has been associated with various genetic conditions, including Neurofibromatosis type 1 (NF1). When moyamoya vasculopathy is present in the context of an associated condition, it is called "moyamoya syndrome," whereas moyamoya pathology in the absence of known associated risk factors is called "moyamoya disease" [47]. Studies have shown that a subset of patients with NF1 experience associated vascular conditions, with moyamoya syndrome representing one of the most common comorbidities. While NF1 and moyamoya syndrome are associated with neurocognitive deficits, very few neuropsychological data ara available for cases of comorbid NF1 and moyamoya syndrome, particularly pre- and post-re-vascularization surgery. To shed light on this topic, DeDios-Sterna and Ventura published in 2019 a single case-study of a bilingual girl of Latin-American descendency with NF1 and moyamoya syndrome, who was assessed pre- (age five years, 9months) and post neurosurgery intervention (age six years, 1month). The pre-neurosurgical cognitive evaluation results documented significant deficits in sustained attention, daily executive functioning, and academic abilities, and the girl met ADHD-combined type criteria. Post- evaluation results revealed generally stable abilities with relative improvements in social, emotional, and behavioral functioning, but a relative decline in visuospatial skills, visual-spatial learning/memory, and executive functioning [48].

Existing literature supports attentional deficits in pMMD, but the clinical presentation of ADHD has rarely been reported. Due to chronic ischemic hypoxic insults to the cerebrum, these patients have poor working memory and experience difficulty sustaining attention, which is thought to be due tohypoperfusion of the frontal lobe. In this sense, Patra and Patnaik reported a clinical case of mental retardation and hyperactivity and inattention five years before the diagnosis of MMD. A definitive diagnosis was made at 11 years of age by means of digital subtraction angiography. The low intellectual functioning and ADHD might have been explained by the chronic cerebral hypoperfusion caused by bilateral internal carotid artery involvement. The neurosurgical procedure had relieved the patient of headaches, but attention deficits and behavioural problemsremained after the operation and required specialized intervention. The decline in the patient's ADHD scores after the neurosurgical procedure might have been due to the persisting cognitive dysfunction caused by the early onset, bilateral arterial involvement, and chronic cerebral hypoperfusion [49].

In rare cases, Moyamoya syndrome is associated with clinical features of movement disorders, like Tourette's syndrome. In this context the first reported clinical case was that of a 5-year-and-9-month-old boy who developed repetitive episodic involuntary winking of the right eye along with ipsilateral shoulder-shrugging movements associated with paroxysmal shouts and loud laughs and punctuated with abusive verbal expressions (coprolalia), progressive regression of verbal and cognitive milestones, emotional lability and aspects of attention deficit hyperkinetic disorder [50]. The child was evaluated by MRI, which showed characteristic ischaemic areas involving the basal ganglia and fronto-parietal cortical regions and the middle cerebral artery territory, predominantly on the left side. Subsequent cerebral angiography revealed extensive stenosis of bilateral (predominantly left-sided) internal cerebral arteries and middle cerebral arteries, with evidence of diffuse leptomeningeal collaterals. The patient was eventually diagnosed with Moyamoya disease with associated Tourette's syndrome. Subsequently, he underwent left-sided superficial temporal artery to middle cerebral artery anastomosis along with encephalo-duro-arterio-myo-synangiosis. Significant clinical-radiological improvement was noted after three months, at which point, the clinical deficiencies had dramatically resolved. There was evidence of an excellent development of direct and indirect surgical collaterals and the left middle cerebral artery territory. The incidence of Moyamoya syndrome associated with intracranial aneurysms ranges from 3% to 14% in adult patients, whereas it is complication rarely reported in children. Noureldine et al. recently reported the first case of an infrequent subarachnoid haemorrhage a child with a ruptured anterior cerebral artery-dissecting aneurysm secondary to a newly discovered, unilateral Moyamoya-like pathology. These authors argued that prompt intervention is essential to exclude the risk of the ruptured aneurysmrebleeding due to persistent hemodynamic stress [51]. Reports on patients with pMMD who present cerebral ischemic complications after intraventricular haemorrhage (IVH) and/or intracerebral bleeding (ICB) are minimal. In this sense, Inoue et al. reported a case of a 7-year-old girl with moyamoya disease with severe cerebral vasospasm and delayed cerebral infarction following an IVH. The authors stressed that, though such cases are rare, the potential for vasospasm-induced cerebral infarction should be considered and, intensive treatment initiated immediately if suspected [52].

We can conclude, based on published evidence, that less neurological insult will lead to better cognitive outcomes. However, the impact of MMD on cognition remains unclear. Even though surgical treatment generally results in positive neurological outcomes, the relationship between the two needs to be investigated. Further clinical studies should focus on a wide range of neuropsychological tests and measurements ofcerebral blood flow and metabolism in large series.

3. MoyaMoya syndrome in adults (aMMD)

Adult MMD patients usually complain of experiencing difficulties in the normal development of their work, typically due to subtle cognitive deficits, but sometimes because of an apparent intellectual disability [53], including occasionally reported cases of progressive dementia associated [54]. Growing interest in patients' neurocognitive profiles can be observed in the scientific literature published in recent years, including those with no neuroradiological evidence of a marked ictus [55–57]. The most recent works suggest that the cognitive impairment in adult MMD is the result of ischemic stroke, but the presence and extent of cognitive decline in asymptomatic patients (those who do not show evidence of ictus, but show some cognitive impairment due to subtle hypoperfusion sustained over years) is an aspect that requires exploration [58]. Some authors have highlighted the absence of a methodological consensus regarding neuropsychological evaluation in MMD as a limitation to definite conclusions [55, 56, 59]. In this sense, the COSMO-JAPAN multicentric prospective study, with 60 adult MMD patients [60] proposed a protocol for cognitive evaluation based on the WAIS-III (intelligence) and WMS-R (memory) tests together with an instrument to measure executive function, such as the FAB (Frontal Assessment Battery), the WCST (Wisconsin Card Classification Test), the Stroop test, the Verbal Fluency Test (FAS) or the TMT A/B (Trail Making Test), and including behavioural scales such as the BDI II (Beck depression scale), the STAI (state-trait anxiety scale), the FrSBe (Frontal behaviour scale), and the WHOQOL26 (a quality of life questionnaire). The results obtained in this study indicated an evident impairment of executive functions, which showedgood correlation with functional neuroimaging data, as a result of vascular involvement (hemodynamic ischemia measured with SPECT at rest) of the anteromedial branches of the anterior cerebral arteries, even in the absence of overt stroke. Functional neuroimaging data has helped to clarify brain-symptomatology relations in MMD. Nakagawara et al. [61] indicated that, even if infarction has not yet occurred, brain dysfunction is associated with persistent hemodynamic compromise in the medial frontal lobes that can be visualized by means of [123I] iomazenil (IMZ) single-photon emission C.T. (SPECT). They highlighted the tremendous potential of this technique as a tool for diagnosing cognitive impairment in adult patients with MMD in whom extensive abnormalities are not revealed by computed tomography (CT) or magnetic resonance imaging (MRI) [61].

In this way, the characterization of the cognitive profile of MMD patients has been the focus of much research in recent years. However, the literature has always indicated that the incidence and severity of cognitive alterations are highly variable among adult patients. In 2008, Karzmark et al. published a survey intended to document more comprehensively the nature of cognitive impairment in moyamoya disease by assessing a larger number of adult cases [57] with a neuropsychological assessment test battery. They demonstrated that the highest rate of impairment corresponded with executive functioning and the lowest rates with memory and perception [62]. Cognitive impairment was present in 31% of the patients, and was severe in 11%. The authors claimedthat MMD can impair cognition in adults, but that the effect is not as severe as in pediatric cases (not the case according to the meta-analyses by Kronenburg et al., which we will address later, which show that the proportion of adult patients with impaired cognitive function matches that of children) [44]. Festa et al. demonstrated that approximately two-thirds of their adult patients (in a pool of 29 patients) exhibited neurocognitive dysfunction [55]. Moreover, a large proportion performed 2 S.D. below the mean on various tests measuring different cognitive domains (29% in processing speed, 31% in verbal memory, 26% in verbal fluency, 25% in executive function). Manual strength and dexterity were also affected in many patients, with impairment detected in 36–58%. The authors suggested that a mechanism of diffuse small vessel disease, perhaps caused by chronic hypoperfusion, could explain the pattern of deficits. Karzmark et al. evaluated another sample of 20 adult MMD patients and observed 67% of them exhibited small T2 hyperintensities in the cerebral subcortical white matter on brain MRI but no evidence of grey-matter damage. Significant cognitive impairment, defined as half of the test scores 1 S.D. below the average mean, was present in 7 patients (23%). Executive functioning, mental efficiency, and word- finding were the ability areas most frequently impaired, whereas memory was relatively intact [57]. Comparable cognitive findings were also observed in the subset of 10 patients (33%) with entirely normal static brain MRI, which lead the authors to conclude that cognitive impairment in MMD can occur in the absence of ischemic stroke as manifested on MRI. As the reader will note, executive dysfunction remains a consistent finding between studies, and Mogensen demonstrated that this impaired executive functioning in adults with MMD is most strongly associated with secondary damage to the brain parenchyma in the form of White Matter Disease (WMD) or cortical stroke [63]. They suggested that increases in global WMD burden were a good indicator of cognitive decline. They also showed that patients with higher baseline CBF tend to have better cognitive functioning.

The treatment for MMD usually consists of surgical revascularization techniques, involving dissecting and re-routing a branch of a superficial artery to a distal branch of another. Revascularization surgery augments cerebral blood flow, and such perfusion augmentation may engender cognitive and neurologic improvement even beyond focal regions of established ischemia. The influence of surgical revascularization treatment on the cognitive status of MMD patients is a subject of debate. This approach is favoured over medical management in children in most cases, but limited data are available regarding the effectiveness of an arterial bypass in adults, especially in terms of cognition improvement. Indeed, there are few published cases reporting neuropsychological status pre- and postrevascularization. Jefferson et al. [64] reported the first case of a 48-year old woman who underwent revascularization following a right hemisphere stroke, and showed a clear temporal relationship between the vascular effects of the bypass procedure and an improvement in neurocognitive status. Preoperative performance in tasks involving visuospatial perception, organization, and construction was generally impaired compared to her estimated premorbid abilities, while postoperative visuospatial performance improved to within a normal range. However, nonverbal visuospatial memory did not return to premorbid levels [64]. Some years after this study, a group of 33 adult patients was assessed pre- and post-surgery in Coutinho's report regarding speech, memory and intellectual processes, in which all the patients underwent stabilization or improvement of physiological symptoms together with significant cognitive improvement after surgery [65].

Another study evaluated a larger group of patients (84) in whom postoperative results were dissapointing: 14% showed significant decline and only 11% an improvement. The majority of patients (75%) displayed neither a significant decline nor an improvement in neurocognitive performance after EC-IC bypass surgery, and similar results were obtained when the analysis was confined to those who underwent unilateral or bilateral revascularization [66]. In light of the fact that adult MMD patients can either improve or decline cognitively after revascularization surgery, Yanagihara et al. [67] emphasized that the intervention boosts cerebral blood flow (CBF) and improves cerebral oxygen metabolism. This cerebral hyperperfusion, which is short-term, can induce a significant increase in ipsilateral CBF that greatly exceed the brain's metabolic needs, thus representing a complication. The authors noted that cerebral hyperperfusion can produce widespread, though minimal, injury to the ipsilateral white matter and cortical regions. In their study of 32 patients, neuropsychological assessments demonstrated cognitive improvement in 31%, no change in 25%, and a decline in 44%. Based on brain perfusion SPECT and symptoms, ten patients were considered to have cerebral hyperperfusion syndrome, and all of these patients exhibited a postoperative decline in cognition.

In summary, acute-stage cerebral hyperperfusion after arterial bypass surgery would seem to impair cognitive function.

On the other hand, an increase in CBF in the chronic stage of cerebral hyperperfusion improves cognitive function in adult patients with symptomatic ischemic MMD [67]. In Moyamoya angioplasty, increased apparent diffusion coefficient (ADC) in frontal white matter (WM) with a normal appearance has been associated with frontal hypoperfusion and executive dysfunction.

Multiple burr-hole surgery enables the revascularization of large frontal areas. In this sense, Calviere et al. recently assessed the effect of such surgery on the ADC and cognitive functions in fourteen adults treated with angioplasty before and six months after the intervention [68]. ADC was obtained from regions of interest located in frontal and posterior (temporo-occipital) normal-appearing WM. Ten patients underwent neuropsychological assessment of executive and attentional functions before and after surgery. The authors concluded that, in MMD adults treated with angioplasty, indirect revascularization by means of burr-hole is followed by a decrease of ADC in normal-appearing frontal WM and may improve some executive functions in the flexibility process. Alterations of ADC may reflect an improvement in cerebral perfusion after surgery. Therefore, the measuring of ADC may be a promising tool to explore potentially reversible microstructural WM damage related to hypoperfusion and cognitive change in aMMD.

In non-surgically treated adult MMD patients with onset of ischemia and stable hemodynamics, the cognitive course remains unclear. In the pool of 70 patients in the study by Miyoshi et al. [69] patients without recurrent ischemic events and no hemodynamic compromise displayed intact cognitive functions two years after the last event. Notably, due to controversy surrounding the surgical option, a large proportion of the patients chose conservative treatment, especially those with hemorrhagic MMD [69]. A study by Su et al. employed the MoCA test to assess cognitive function in 26 adult patients with hemorrhagic MMD who received no surgical revascularization, and observed Mild Cognitive Impairment (MCI) after two years in all 26 [70]. These patients obtained significant decreases in all MoCA subscores ($P = 0.000$) regarding delayed recall, visual space and executive function. However, in a longitudinal case series of adults who had suffered stroke secondary to MMD, stroke recovery was good providing the patient was treated transdisciplinary for 3-4 months (as well as being young and healthy and highly functional prior to the stroke) [71]. The functionality of the patients seems to be more critical than supposed. In Araki's [56] study, the ten patients, were divided into those without difficulties maintaining social independence, with higher educational background, better socioeconomic status, no need for public support, and those who had social independence issues and were socioeconomically disadvantaged. The study found subtle impairments in intelligence and working memory in all the sample. However, frontal lobe functions were primarily affected in adult MMD patients with a social independence problem, even if brain imaging techniques did not reveal noticeable abnormalities [56].

All the questions mentioned above were studied in the meta-analysies of cognitive functions performed by Kronenburg et al. [44], and which included 17 studies (11 studies reporting on 281 children, six on 153 adults). Regarding the adult samples, the median percentage with impaired cognition was as high as 31% (range, 0% to 69%), their median I.Q. scores were within the normal range (95; in a range of 94 to 99), and the median z-scores of cognitive domains were between –0.9 and –0.4, with many of them being affected. The highest median percentage of impaired function was detected for domain attention and executive functions. In a previous review, these authors had suggested that cognition is affected more frequently in children than in adults, reporting intelligence to be impaired in children, and executive functions to be impaired in adults. However, in this systematic review (more detailed and complete), they concluded that the proportion of adult patients with cognitive function impairment is as large as in children. Moreover, the authors could not identify specific determinants of cognitive deficits and deterioration, and urged for further studies to examine such questions, as well as the influence of revascularization treatment on cognitive functioning. The general recommendation for the future was extensive prospective studies using a standardized battery of neuropsychological tests to determine the severity of cognitive impairment and the domains affected, with the inclusion of information on school-level and performance, and on work status, since it reflects functionality rather than deficits [44].

Recent reports (following this metaanalysies) have followed in the same direction regarding the alteration of attention and executive functions. Jia-Bin et al. discovered that, in a sample of 34 MMD patients, one group performed significantly worse than controls in the Symbol Digit Modalities Test ($z = 4.555$, $P < 0.001$) and The Trail-Making Test Part B ($z = 3.953$, $P < 0.001$). An impairment of memory measured through the long-term delayed recall of the Auditory Verbal Learning Test ($P < 0.001$) was also observed [72]. A neurocognitive evaluation case report by Indorewalla et al. [73] showed a lateralized profile and impairments in simple auditory attention, processing speed, working memory, verbal learning, verbal fluency, and speeded fine-motor dexterity.

Importantly, the latest studies about cognition in adult MMD consider other factors, like gender and clinical subtypes [73]. Shi et al. [74] studied a sample of 49 patients divided into 12 hemorrhagic subjects and 37 with ischemia and compared them with healthy controls. All the patients displayed comprehensive cognitive impairment affecting the domain of memory (prospective and retrospective memory), verbal fluency and executive functions (measured with the Stroop test) [74]. They also showed a pattern of attention significantly different from controls (including impairment in the Trail Making Test-A). Interestingly, female patients performed better than male patients, showing significant differences in forward and immediate memory, Stroop and Wisconsin Card Sorting Test. Another intringuing result was that the hemorrhagic patients, fared poorer in the dimension of prospective and retrospective memory than their ischemic counterparts. Besides, prospective and retrospective memory, attention and executive functions were moderately correlated. A recent study exploring the clinical features of MMD sufferers compared 19 patients with a history of cerebral infarction with 21 asymptomatic patients (plus 20 healthy controls matched for age, sex, and years of education). Detailed neuropsychological testing revealed varying degrees of decline in intelligence, spatial imagination, verbal working memory and computational ability (simple and complex subtraction) in asymptomatic patients compared to normal controls. Patients with cerebral infarction showed more severe impairment in complex arithmetic and short-term memory than those without symptoms. In conclusion, the authors suggested that asymptomatic patients can present various cognitive impairments that precedes the onset of clinical signs such as cerebral infarction, which may be a long-term complication of conservative treatment. Future research should address in depth the distinctive profile of MMD patients according to their neurological clinical status, the influence of gender and educational level on their cognition, and the importance of functional independence in their rehabilitation.

Moyamoya disease and atherosclerotic cerebrovascular disease are chronic ischemic diseases with similar consequences in the form of vascular cognitive impairment. The aim of the study conducted by Su et al. [75] was to investigate the patterns of microstructural damage associated with vascular cognitive impairment in the two diseases in a sample of 34 patients with MMD (mean age 43.9),

27 patients with atherosclerotic cerebovascular disease (mean age: 44.6), and 31 normal controls (mean age 43.6) from Huashan Hospital of Fudan University, in China. Cognitive function was assessed using the Mini-Mental State Examination, long-term delayed recall of the Auditory Verbal Learning Test, the Trail-Making Test Part B, and the Symbol Digit Modalities Test. Single-photon emission-computed tomography was used to examine cerebral perfusion. Voxel-based morphometry and tract-based spatial statistics were performed to identify regions of gray matter atrophy and white matter deterioration in patients and controls. The results demonstrated that the severity of cognitive impairment in the two diseases was similar in all the tested domains. Both patients with MMD and those with atherosclerotic cerebrovascular disease exhibited altered supratentorial hemodynamics; gray matter atrophy was evident in the middle cingulate cortex and parts of the frontal gyrus in both groups, but was generally more severe and more diffuse in those with MMD. White matter deterioration was significant in both diseases, in the genu and body of the corpus callosum, the anterior and superior corona radiation, and the posterior thalamic radiation, but was more diffuse and more severe in MMD. Vascular cognitive impairment was associated with regional microstructural damage, with a potential link between gray and white matter damage being highlighted [75].

A last point of interest to mention is that MMD patients sometimes present with cognitive dysfunction and psychiatric or neuropsychiatric symptoms. In 1991, McDade described a rare case of schizophrenia in a 19-years-old boy with MMD [76]. Nagata et al. reported the case of a 50-year-old man who suffered from irritability and agitation that affected his work and relationships after developing a right ipsilateral frontal lobe infarction as a result of MMD [77]. Zalonis et al. described a case of a middle-aged woman who suffered intraventricular haemorrhages due to MMD. Initially, she presented psychiatric symptoms (mood disorder, irritability, or agitation) that did not respond to treatment. Neuropsychological assessment revealed underlying significant cognitive deficits, mostly of complex attention and speed of information processing, visuospatial and constructional abilities, verbal and nonverbal memory, and executive functions. These deficits continued to be present or had improved slightly when follow-up was carried out [78]. Hong et al. [79] described a patient (a 22-year-old, right-handed woman) who presented with transient cortical blindness, anosognosia, and global transitory amnesia associated with MMD. The woman completely denied blindness and recent memory disturbances with confabulation. This case report demonstrated that MMD can manifest itself in transient posterior circulation symptoms in the form of Dide-Botcazo syndrome [55]. Of the 29 adult American MMD patients included in the Festa et al. study, 36% were found to suffer mild depression and 28% to suffer moderate-to-severe depression, as measured by the Beck Depression Inventory (BDI) [55]. In their 2008 study, Karzmak et al. reported five patients with mild depression, and two patients with moderate depression, and later (in their 2012 study) reported clinically significant emotional distress (depression and/or anxiety) in (37% of their cohort) [62]. In summary, although exclusively psychiatric presentations of MMD in adults are exceedingly rare in the literature, complaints of depression or anxiety often do accompany new focal neurological symptoms, and psychosis can indeed occur. In this way, MMD carries with the risk of misdiagnosis as an affective or psychotic disorder. Transient ischemic events may be mistaken for anxiety and panic disorder, and so there is a call for careful screening of precipitating triggers and characterization of symptoms. When a MMD patient shows psychiatric clinical signs, in the absence of a family history (particularly one of psychotic illness), in combination with atypical features (age at onset, visual hallucinations), a neurological investigation is advised, namely MRI or M.R. angiography rather than C.T.

screening. In the cases of new psychiatric symptoms in patients with diagnosed MMD, repeated neuroimaging is called for to rule out further ischemia [80].

Since the main neurovascular alterations of MMD tend to affect fronto-temporal areas, we propose that any neuropsychological evaluation shouldinclude the study of executive functions (working memory, processing speed, sustained and divided attention), intelligence (I.Q., especially in pMMD), verbal memory (including recognition memory) and visual memory. Given the variety of clinical and cognitive symptoms and different forms of presentation and evolution of MMD, we recommend a baseline and neuropsychological follow-up of all patients with a suspected or definitive clinical diagnosis of MMD.

Author details

Raúl Espert* and Marien Gadea
Psychobiology Department, University of Valencia, Valencia, Spain

*Address all correspondence to: raul.espert@uv.es

References

[1] Suzuki J, Takaku A. Cerebrovascular 'moyamoya' disease showing abnormal net-like vessels in base of the brain. Archives of Neurology. 1969; 20: 288-299. DOI:10.1001/archneur.1969.00480090076012.

[2] Takeuchi K, Shimizu K. Hypogenesis of bilateral internal carotid arteries. No To Shinkei. 1957; 9: 37-43. DOI: 10.12691/ajmcr-2-5-5

[3] Chiu D, Shedden P, Bratina P, Grotta JC. Clinical features of moyamoya disease in the United States. Stroke. 1998; 29: 1347-1351. DOI: 10.1161/01.str.29.7.1347.

[4] Zhang H, Zheng L and Feng L: Epidemiology, diagnosis and treatment of moyamoya disease (Review). Experimental and Therapeutic Medicine. 2019; 17: 1977-1984. https://doi.org/10.3892/etm.2019.7198

[5] Baba T, Houkin K, Kuroda S. Novel epidemiological features of moyamoya disease. Journal of Neurology Neurosurgery and Psychiatry. 2008; 79: 900-4. DOI: 10.1136/jnnp.2007.130666.

[6] Wakai K, Tamakoshi A, Ikezaki K, Fukui M, Kawamura T, Aoki R, et. al. Epidemiological features of moyamoya disease in Japan: findings from a nationwide survey. Clinical Neurology and Neurosurgery. 1997; 99 (Suppl 2): S1-5. DOI: 10.1016/s0303-8467(97)00031-0.

[7] Yonekawa Y, Ogata N, Kaku Y, Taub E, Imhof HG. Moyamoya disease in Europe, past and present status. Clinical Neurology and Neurosurgery. 1997; 99 (Suppl 2): S58-60. DOI: 10.1016/s0303-8467(97)00042-5.

[8] Uchino K, Johnston SC, Becker KJ, Tirschwell DL. Moyamoya disease in Washington State and California. Neurology 2005; 65: 956-8. DOI: 10.1016/s0303-8467(97)00042-5.

[9] Shoubhi B, Digish S. A rare cause of seizures in children: "Moyamoya disease". Medical Journal of Dr. D.Y. Patil University. 2016; 19 (3): 393-396. DOI: 10.4103/0975-2870.182519

[10] Scott RM, Smith ER. Moyamoya disease and Moyamoya syndrome. New England Journal of Medicine. 2009; 360: 1226-37. DOI: 10.1056/NEJMra0804622

[11] Nagiub M, Allarakhia EI. Pediatric Moyamoya disease. American Journal of Case Reports. 2013; 14: 134-138. DOI: 10.12659/AJCR.889170

[12] Smith JL. Understanding and treating moyamoya disease in children. Neurosurgery Focus. 2009; 26 (4): 1-11. DOI: 10.3171.2000.01.FOCUS08306

[13] Maki Y, Enomoto T. Moyamoya disease. Child's Nervous System. 1988;4:204-212.

[14] Wang CX, Wang QY, Zhao YM, Zhou M, Chen XX, Zhang RY. Causes, clinical and imaging characteristics of moyamoya disease in children. Biomedical Research. 2018; 29 (6): 1154-1159. DOI: 10.4066/biomedicalresearch.29-17-2904

[15] Papavasiliou A, Bazigou-Fotopoulou H, Ikeda H. Familial Moyamoya disease in two European children. Journal of Child Neurology. 2007; 22:1371-1376. DOI: 10.1177/0883073807307101.

[16] Piao J, Wu W, Yang Z, Yu J. Research Progress of Moyamoya Disease in Children. International Journal of Medical Sciences. 2015, 12: 566-575. DOI: 10.7150/ijms.11719.

[17] Hsu YH, Kuo MF, Hua MS, Yang CC: Selective neuropsychological impairments and related clinical factors in children with moyamoya disease of the transient ischemic attack type.

Child's Nervous System. 2014; 30: 441-447. DOI: 10.1007/s00381-013-2271-9

[18] Imaizumi C, Imaizumi T, Osawa M, Fukuyama Y, Takeshita M: Serial intelligence test scores in pediatric moyamoya disease. Neuropediatrics. 1999; 30: 294-299. DOI: 10.1055/s-2007-973508.

[19] Imaizumi T, Hayashi K, Saito K, Osawa M, Fukuyama Y: Long-term outcomes of pediatric moyamoya disease monitored to adulthood. Pediatric Neurology. 1998; 18: 321-325. DOI: 10.1016/s0887-8994(97)00209-9

[20] Hsu YH, Kuo MF, Hua MS, Yang CC: Selective neuropsychological impairments and related clinical factors in children with moyamoya disease of the transient ischemic attack type. Child's Nervous System. 2014; 30: 441-447. DOI: 10.1007/s00381-013-2271-9

[21] Shim KW, Park EK, Kim, JS, Kim DS: Cognitive Outcome of Pediatric Moyamoya Disease. Journal of Korean Neurosurgery Society. 2015; 57 (6): 440-444. http://dx.doi.org/10.3340/jkns.2015.57.6.440

[22] Ishii R, Takeuchi S, Ibayashi K, Tanaka R: Intelligence in children with moyamoya disease: evaluation after surgical treatments with special reference to changes in cerebral blood flow. Stroke. 1984; 15 : 873-877. DOI: 10.1161/01.str.15.5.873.

[23] Matsushima Y, Aoyagi M, Masaoka H, Suzuki R, Ohno K: Mental outcome following encephaloduroarteriosynangiosis in children with moyaamoya disease with the onset earlier than 5 years of age. Child's Nervous System. 1990; 6: 440-443. DOI: 10.1007/BF00302089

[24] Rafay MF, Armstrong D, Dirks P, MacGregor DL, deVeber G. Patterns of Cerebral Ischemia in Children With Moyamoya. Pediatric Neurology. 2015; 52 (1): 65-72. https://doi.org/10.1016/j.pediatrneurol.2014.10.007Wnag

[25] Imaizumi T, Hayashi K, Saito K, Osawa M, Fukuyama Y: Long-term outcomes of pediatric moyamoya disease monitored to adulthood. Pediatric Neurology. 1998; 18: 321-325. DOI: 10.1016/s0887-8994(97)00209-9.

[26] Imaizumi C, Imaizumi T, Osawa M, Fukuyama Y, Takeshita M: Serial intelligence test scores in pediatric moyamoya disease. Neuropediatrics. 1999; 30: 294-299. DOI: 10.1055/s-2007-973508.

[27] Ishikawa T, Houkin K, Kamiyama H, Abe H: Effects of surgical revascularization on outcome of patients with pediatric moyamoya disease. Stroke. 1997; 28: 1170-1173. https://doi.org/10.1161/01.STR.28.6.1170

[28] Karasawa J, Touho H, Ohnishi H, Miyamoto S, Kikuchi H: Long-term follow-up study after extracranial-intracranial bypass surgery for anterior circulation ischemia in childhood moyamoya disease. Journal of Neurosurgery. 1992; 77: 84-89. https://doi.org/10.3171/jns.1992.77.1.0084

[29] Miyamoto S, Akiyama Y, Nagata I, Karasawa J, Nozaki K, Hashimoto N, et al.: Long-term outcome after STA-MCA anastomosis for moyamoya disease. Neurosurgical Focus. 1998; 5: e5. https://doi.org/10.3171/foc.1998.5.5.8

[30] Kim SK, Cho BK, Hoon J, Lee JY, Chae JH, Kim KJ, Hwang YS, Kim IO, Lee DS, Lee J, Wang KC. Pediatric moyamoya disease: An analysis of 410 consecutive cases. Annals of Neurology, 2010; 68(1):92-101. doi: 10.1002/ana.21981.

[31] Titsworth WL, Scott M, Smith ER. National Analysis of 2454 Pediatric Moyamoya Admissions and the Effect of Hospital Volume on Outcomes Stroke.

2016;47:1303-1311. DOI: 10.1161/STROKEAHA.115.01216

[32] Tho-Calvi SC, Thompson D, Saunders D, Agrawal S, Basu A, Chitre M, Chow G, Gibbon F, Hart A, Tallur KK, Kirkham F, Kneen R, McCullagh H, Mewasingh L, Vassallo G, Vijayakumar K, Wraige E, Yeo TH, Ganesan V. Clinical features, course, and outcomes of a UK cohort of pediatric moyamoya. Neurology. 2018; 90 (9). DOI: https://doi.org/10.1212/WNL.0000000000005026

[33] Cooper AN, Anderson V, Hearps S, Greenham M, Hunt RW, Mackay MT, Monagle P, Gordon AL. The Pediatric Stroke Outcome Measure. A predictor of outcome following arterial ischemic stroke. Neurology. 2018; 90 (5). DOI https://doi.org/10.1212/WNL.0000000000004906

[34] Funaki T, Takahashi JC, Miyamoto S. Late Cerebrovascular Events and Social Outcome after Adolescence: Long-term Outcome of Pediatric Moyamoya Disease. Neurologia Medico-Chirurgica (Tokyo). 2018; 15;58(6):240-246. DOI: 10.2176/nmc.ra.2018-0026.

[35] Appireddy R, Ranjan M, Durafourt BA, Riva-Cambrin J, Hader WJ, Adelson PD. Surgery for Moyamoya Disease in Children. J Child Neurol. 2019 Aug; 34(9):517-529. DOI: 10.1177/0883073819844854.

[36] Piao J, Wu W, Yang Z, Yu J. Research Progress of Moyamoya Disease in Children. International Journal of Medical Sciences. 2015; 12 (7): 566-575. DOI: 10.7150/ijms.11719

[37] Kim W, Lee EY, Park SE, Park EK. Kim JS, Kim DS, Shim KW. Neuropsychological impacts of indirect revascularization for pediatric moyamoya disease. Child's Nervous System. 2018; 34(6):1199-1206 DOI: 10.1007/s00381-018-3804-z

[38] Williams TS, Westmacott R, Dlamini N, Granite L, Dirks P, Askalan R, Macgregor D, Moharir M, Deveber G. Intellectual ability and executive function in pediatric moyamoya vasculopathy. Developmental Medicine & Child Neurology. 2012; 54(1):30-7. DOI: 10.1111/j.1469-8749.2011.04144.x.

[39] Gutiérrez-Martignon, M, Prieto-Corona, B, Bernal, J, Rodríguez-Camacho, M, Salvador, J, García, A, Velasco, E, Grijalva, I, Armejo L. Cognitive outcome of a pediatric stroke case: Moyamoya disease. Panamerican Journal of Neuropsychology. 2020; 14 (2): 71-82. DOI: 10.7714/CNPS/14.2.301

[40] Ball AJ, Steinberg GK, Elbers J. Quality of Life in Pediatric Moyamoya Disease. Pediatric Neurology. 2016; 63: 60-65. https://doi.org/10.1016/j.pediatrneurol.2016.06.012

[41] Gupta SK, Agarwal A, and Mohanty M. Moyamoya Disease: Assessment of Neurological and neuropsychological outcome Following Revascularization Procedures. Journal of Neurological Surgery Part B: Skull Base 2013; 74(S 01): A179. DOI: 10.1055/s-0033-1336302

[42] Nehra A, Kaur H. Moyamoya Disease: a ray of hope from a psychosocial perspective. Annals of Neurosciences. 2015; 22 (2): 121-124. DOI: 10.5214/ans.0972.7531.221212

[43] Cusin-Lamônica DA, da Costa Ribeiro C, Duarte Pinto Ferraz PM, Merighi Tabaquim ML. Moyamoya disease: impact on the performance of oral and written language. CoDAS. 2016; 28(5):661-665. DOI: 10.1590/2317-1782/20162016010.

[44] Kronenbourg A, van den Berg E, van Schooneveld MM, Braun KPJ, Dios L, van der Zwan A, Klijna CJM. Cognitive Functions in Children and Adults with Moyamoya Vasculopathy:

A Systematic Review and Meta-Analysis. Journal of Stroke. 2018;20(3):332-341. https://doi.org/10.5853/jos.2018.01550

[45] Kazumata K, Tokairin K, Sugiyama T, Ito M, Uchino H, Osanai T, Kawabori M, Nakayama N, Houkin K. Association of cognitive function with cerebral blood flow in children with moyamoya disease. Journal of Neurosurgery. 2019; DOI link: https://doi.org/10.3171/2019.7.PEDS19312

[46] Li J, Liu X, Zhang D, Zhang Y, Wang R, Yuan J and Zhao J. Cognitive Performance Profile in Pediatric Moyamoya Disease Patients and Its Relationship With Regional Cerebral Blood Perfusion. 2019. Frontiers in Neurology; 10:1308. DOI: 10.3389/fneur.2019.01308

[47] Scott RM, Smith, ER. Moyamoya disease and moyamoya syndrome. The New England Journal of Medicine. 2009; 360(12), 1226-1236. DOI: 10.1056/NEJMra0804622.

[48] DeDios-Sterna S, Ventura LM. A pediatric case of NF1 and moyamoya syndrome: neuropsychological evaluation pre- and post-EDAS. Applied Neuropsychology (Child). 2019; DOI: 10.1080/21622965.2019.1665292

[49] Patra S, Patnaik A. Pediatric moyamoya disease presenting as attention deficit hyperactivity disorder: Time to pay attention. Indian Journla of Psychiatry. 2019;61(5):544-545. DOI: 10.4103/psychiatry.IndianJPsychiatry_403_18.

[50] Bose R, Banerjee AD. Paediatric Moyamoya Disease and Tourette's Syndrome: An Unusual Association Responding Favourably to Direct and Indirect Cerebral Revascularisation Surgery. Pediatric Neurosurgery. 2019;54:436-440 https://doi.org/10.1159/000503114

[51] Noureldine MHA, Saikali, I, Nassif A., Chahinian R, Sweid A, Kikano R, Mawad M. Pediatric Moyamoya Presenting as a Subarachnoid Hemorrhage from a Ruptured Anterior Cerebral Artery Aneurysm. World Neurosurgery. 2020; 134: 123-127. https://doi.org/10.1016/j.wneu.2019.10.157

[52] Inoue K, Shimokawa S, Yoshioka F, Ogata A, Masuoka J, Abe T. A case of pediatric moyamoya disease with severe cerebral vasospasm and delayed cerebral infarction following an intraventricular hemorrhage. Childs Nervous System. 2020 Jul 14. DOI: 10.1007/s00381-020-04769-2.

[53] Espert R, Gadea M, Aliño M, Oltra-Cucarella J, Perpiñá C. Enfermedad de moyamoya: aspectos clínicos, neurorradiológicos, neuropsicolológicos y genéticos. Revista de Neurología. 2018; 66 (S01): 57-64 DOI: 10.33588/rn.66S01.2017526

[54] Castañeda MA, Peña CS, Cabillas MLL. Enfermedad de Moyamoya: Cefalea crónica y demencia progresiva asociadas a infartos cerebrales multiples. Revista de Neuropsiquiatría. 2019; 82(4):285-292. DOI: 10.20453/rnp.v82i4.3650

[55] Festa JR, Schwarz LR, Pliskin N, Cullum CM, Lacritz L, Charbel FT, et al. Neurocognitive dysfunction in adult MMD disease. Journal of Neurology. 2010; 257: 806-15. DOI: 10.1007/s00415-009-5424-8

[56] Araki Y, Takagi Y, Ueda K, Ubukata S, Ishida J, Funaki T, et al. Cognitive function of patients with adult moyamoya disease. Journal of stroke and cerebrovascular diseases. 2014; 23(7): 1789-1794 DOI: 10.1016/j.jstrokecerebrovasdis.2014.04.032.

[57] Karzmark P, Zeifert PD, Bell-Stephens TE, Steinberg GK, Dorfman LJ. Neurocognitive impairment in adults with MMD disease without stroke. Neurosurgery

2012; 70: 634-8. DOI: 10.1227/NEU.0b013e3182320d1a.

[58] He S, Duan R, Liu Z, Yuan L, Li T, Tan C, Shao J, Qin S, Wang R. Characteristics of cognitive impairment in adult asymptomatic MMD disease. BMC Neurology. 2020; 20: 322. https://doi.org/10.1186/s12883-020-01898-8

[59] Weinberg DG, Rahme RJ, Aoun SG, Batjer HH, Bendok BB. Moyamoya disease: functional and neurocognitive outcomes in the pediatric and adult populations. Neurosurgery Focus. 2011; 30: E21. DOI: 10.3171/2011.3.FOCUS1150

[60] Takagi Y, Miyamoto S, COSMO-Japan Study Group. Cognitive dysfunction survey of the Japanese patients with MMD disease (COSMO-JAPAN Study): study protocol. Neurologia Medico-Chirurgica (Tokyo) 2015; 55: 199-203. DOI: 10.2176/nmc.ra.2014-0326.

[61] Nakagawara J, Osato T, Kamiyama K, Honjo K, Sugio H, Fumoto K, et al. Diagnostic imaging of higher brain dysfunction in patients with adult MMD disease using statistical imaging analysis for [123I] iomazenil single-photon emission computed tomography. Neurologia Medico-Chirurgica (Tokyo) 2012; 52: 318-26. DOI: 10.2176/nmc.52.318

[62] Karzmark P, Zeifert PD, Tan S. Dorfman LJ, Bell-Stephens TE, Steinberg GK. Effect of moyamoya disease on neuropsychological functioning in adults. Neurosurgery. 2008; 62:1048-1052 DOI:10.1227/01.neu.0000325866.29634.4c.

[63] Mogensen MA, Karzmark P, Zeifert PD, Rosenberg J, Marks M, Steinberg GK, Dorfman LJ. Neuroradiologic Correlates of Cognitive Impairment in Adult Moyamoya Disease. AJNR American Journal of Neuroradiology. 2012; 33:721-25 DOI: https://doi.org/10.3174/ajnr.A2852

[64] Jefferson AL, Glosser G, Detre JA, Sinson G, Liebeskind DS. Neuropsychological and perfusion MR imaging correlates of revascularization in a case of moyamoya syndrome. American Journal of Neuroradiology. 2006; 27(1): 98-100. PMID: 16418365 PMCID: PMC2721464

[65] Coutinho, VT. Cognitive Improvement After Microsurgical Revascularization for the Treatment of Moyamoya Disease [thesis]. North Florida: UNF Graduate Theses and Dissertations. 505. 2014. https://digitalcommons.unf.edu/etd/505

[66] Zeifert PD, Karzmark P, Bell-Stephens TE, Steinberg GK, Dorfman L. Neurocognitive performance after cerebral revascularization in adult moyamoya disease. Stroke. 2017; 48:1514-1517. DOI: 10.1161/STROKEAHA.116.016028

[67] Yanagihara W, Chida K, Kobayashi M, Kubo Y, Yoshida K, Terasaki K, Ogasawara K. Impact of cerebral blood flow changes due to arterial bypass surgery on cognitive function in adult patients with symptomatic ischemic moyamoya disease. Journal of Neurosurgery. 2019; 131:1716-1724. DOI: https://doi.org/10.3171/2018.7.JNS18149

[68] Calviere, L., Loubiere, P., Planton, M. et al. Decreased frontal white-matter diffusion and improved cognitive flexibility after burr-hole surgery in moyamoya angiopathy. BMC Neurology. 2020. 20: 30 https://doi.org/10.1186/s12883-020-1614-x

[69] Miyoshi K, Chida K, Kobayashi M, Kubo Y, Yoshida K, Terasaki K, Ogasawara K. Two-year clinical, cerebral hemodynamic, and cognitive outcomes of adult patients undergoing

medication alone for symptomatically ischemic moyamoya disease without cerebral misery perfusion: a prospective cohort study. Neurosurgery. 2019; 84 (6): 1233. DOI: 10.1093/neuros/nyy234.

[70] Su SH, Hai J, Zhang L, Yu F, Wu YF. Assessment of cognitive function in adult patients with hemorrhagic moyamoya disease who received no surgical revascularization. European Journal of Neurology. 2013; 20: 1081-1087. DOI: 10.1111/ene.12138.

[71] Perna R, McGee J. Case series of adults with Moyamoya-related stroke and rehabilitation outcomes. Biology and Medicine Case Report. 2017; 1(1):24-26. DOI: 10.35841/biology-medicine.1.1.24-26

[72] Jia-Bin S, Xi SD, Zhou SY, Zhang X, Jiang SH, Xu B, Chen L, Lei Y, MD, Gao C, Gu YX. Microstructural damage pattern of vascular cognitive impairment: a comparison between moyamoya disease and cerebrovascular atherosclerotic disease. Neural Regeneration Research. 2019; 14 (5): 858-867. DOI:10.4103/1673-5374.249234.

[73] Indorewalla K, McArdle M, Tomlinson E, Piryatinsky I. Neuropsychological profile associated with MMD disease: A case report. NeuroRehabilitation. 2020; 46 (4): 603-611 DOI: 10.3233/NRE-192903.

[74] Shi Z, Wen Y-J, Huang Z, Yu LB, Zhang D. Different aspects of cognitive function in adult patients with moyamoya disease and its clinical subtypes. Stroke & Vascular Neurology. 2020: 5; e000309. DOI:10.1136/svn-2019-000309

[75] Su JB, Xi SD, Zhou SY, Zhang X, Jiang SH, Xu B, Chen L, Lei Y, Gao C, Gu YX. Microstructural damage pattern of vascular cognitive impairment: a comparison between moyamoya disease and cerebrovascular atherosclerotic disease. Neural Regeneration Research. 2019;14(5):858-867. DOI: 10.4103/1673-5374.249234.

[76] McDade G. Symptomatic schizophrenia with moya-moya disease. Behavioral Neurology. 1991;4(1):25-8. DOI: 10.3233/BEN-1991-4103.

[77] Nagata T, Harada D, Aoki K, et al. Effectiveness of carbamazepine for benzodiazepine-resistant impulsive aggression in a patient with frontal infarctions. Psychiatry and Clinical Neuroscience. 2007; 61:695-697. DOI: 10.1111/j.1440-1819.2007.01737.x.

[78] Zalonis I, Christidi F, Kararizou E, Triantafyllou NI, Spengos K, Vassilopoulos D. Cognitive deficits presenting as psychiatric symptoms in a patient with moyamoya disease. Psychological Reports. 2010; 107, 3: 727-732. DOI: 10.2466/02.13.15.22.PR0.107.6.727-732.

[79] Hong JY, Na SJ, Shin JW, Kim HS, Kim WC, et al. Moyamoya disease presenting as transient amnesia with cortical blindness. Journal of Neurosonology and Neuroimaging. 2019; 11(2): 169-172. DOI: https://doi.org/10.31728/jnn.2019.00067

[80] Richards M, Grzenda A, Nelson E, Gitlin M. Psychiatric Comorbidity in Moyamoya Disease and Preliminary Guidelines For Treatment. American Journal of Psychiatry. 2019; 176:4. https://doi.org/10.1176/appi.ajp.2018.18040404

Section 5

Perioperative Anesthetic Management of Moyamoya Disease

Chapter 5

Perioperative Considerations for Revascularization and Non-Revascularization Surgeries in Moyamoya Disease

Muhammad Jaffar Khan, Jazib Hassan, Sumayya Aboobacker, Tarek Tageldin, Jafar Faraj and Mohamed El-Arref

Abstract

Moyamoya disease is a rare, progressive cerebrovascular occlusive disease; characterized by narrowing of the distal internal carotid arteries and their branches. The incidence is high in East Asians and most commonly presents in the first and fourth decade of life. Its symptoms are headaches, seizures, transient neurological deficits, and cognitive decline. Medical management is based on treating the symptoms and includes antiplatelet and anti-seizure medications. Surgical revascularization is the mainstay of treatment. Unique pathophysiology of moyamoya disease necessitates neuro-anesthesiologists to formulate an individualized plan perioperatively. The overriding goal of perioperative anesthetic management of moyamoya disease is to ensure optimal cerebral perfusion and protection. Maintenance of normotension, normocarbia, normo-oxygenation, normothermia, and euvolemia is the cornerstone during the perioperative period. Perioperative adequate analgesia is crucial to prevent cerebral ischemia and allows close neurological monitoring. This chapter reviews perioperative anesthetic management of patients with moyamoya disease.

Keywords: moyamoya disease, perioperative consideration, anesthetic management, indocyanine green, total intravenous anesthesia, scalp nerve block, special considerations in non-revascularization surgery

1. Introduction

Moyamoya disease is a unique cerebrovascular condition that is characterized by slowly progressive narrowing of the terminal portion of the internal carotid artery and its proximal branches. The name of this disease is derived from the dilated and fragile distal collateral vessels, which develop over time and demonstrate a characteristic "puff of smoke" appearance (see **Figure 1**) on cerebral angiography [1, 2]. On the other hand, moyamoya syndrome is traditionally considered in patients who have the characteristics vasculopathy and associated conditions, such as sickle cell disease or neurofibromatosis [3]. The incidence of moyamoya disease (MMD) is

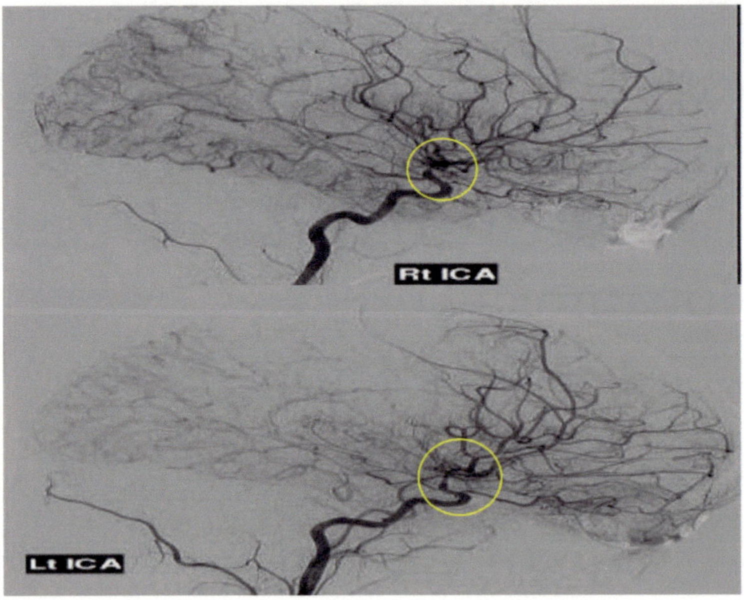

Figure 1.
Bilateral internal carotid artery narrowing at the bifurcation with characteristic "puff of smoke" collateral circulation on cerebral angiography. Picture courtesy of Dr. Jafar (Hamad Medical Corporation).

high in East Asia, and familial links account for 15% of the patients. It has a bimodal distribution which includes two peaks of age distribution at 5 years and 40 years [4, 5]. The pathophysiology of MMD is not a well-studied entity. However, genetic acquired, and environmental factors have been ascribed. Mutation analysis of the RNF213 gene showed a strong correlation with MMD [6]. Histologically, MMD results from fibro-cellular thickening of the intimal layer of the cerebral arteries that progress to vessel narrowing and secondary vascular proliferation. Traditionally, moyamoya disease manifests itself bilaterally; these stenotic lesions are progressive; and thus, the patients present for bilateral procedures. Classically, MMD can present as transient ischemic attacks (TIA), ischemic or hemorrhagic stroke, headache, epilepsy, and cognitive dysfunction with the occurrence of each symptoms varying depending on the age of the patient. Diagnostic criteria for MMD have been established by the Research Committee on Spontaneous Occlusions of the Circle of Willis (Moyamoya Disease) of the Ministry of Health and Welfare of Japan [7] and are presented in **Table 1**. In 1969, Takaku and Suzuki developed angiographic staging to document the progression of MMD [8] as demonstrated in **Table 2**. Medical management is aimed at reducing the risk of stroke or controlling seizures [4, 9]. Aspirin or other antiplatelet drugs are recommended to prevent strokes whereas, anti-seizure drugs should be prescribed if the patient has a seizure disorder. The definitive treatment is surgical, which involves direct or indirect revascularization techniques, or a combination of both may be used. Indirect procedures include encephaloduroarteriosynangiosis (EDAS) or encephalomyossynangiosis. In a direct revascularization procedure, the superficial temporal artery of the scalp is anastomosed directly to a cerebral artery (middle cerebral artery) to increase blood flow to the brain [10, 11]. The perioperative management of MMD presents unique challenges and mandates individualized perioperative strategy [12]. In this chapter, we review the perioperative anesthetic considerations for revascularization and non-revascularization surgery in MMD patients with relevance to the current evidence base and clinical guidelines. It is aimed to be a comprehensive review for residents and fellows training in the field of neuroanaesthesia.

Criteria 1. Cerebral Angiography—must demonstrate at least three of the following	i. Stenosis or occlusion of the distal internal carotid artery (ICA) or proximal portions of the anterior cerebral artery (ACA) or middle cerebral artery (MCA) ii. Abnormal vascular networks near the stenotic lesions iii. Bilateral findings
Criteria 2. If MRI and MRA demonstrate all of the following criteria, angiography can be deferred	i. Stenosis or occlusion of the distal ICA or proximal portions of the ACA or MCA ii. Abnormal vascular networks in the basal ganglia iii. Bilateral findings
Criteria 3. Exclusion of the following	i. Atherosclerosis ii. Autoimmune disease iii. Meningitis iv. Brain tumor v. Down's syndrome vi. Von Recklinghausen's disease vii. Head injury viii. Cerebrovascular lesions after head irradiation

Table 1.
Diagnostic criteria for Moyamoya disease [7].

Stage 1	• Stenosis of suprasellar ICA, usually bilateral
Stage 2	• Development of moyamoya vessels at base of brain
Stage 3	• Increasing ICA stenosis and prominence of moyamoya vessels
Stage 4	• Entire circle of Willis and PCAs occluded, extracranial collaterals start to appear, moyamoya vessels begin to diminish
Stage 5	• Further progression of stage 4 with progressive reduction of moyamoya vessels
Stage 6	• Complete absence of moyamoya vessels and major cerebral arteries

Table 2.
Angiographic staging for progression of MMD [8].

2. Perioperative anesthetic consideration for revascularization or intracranial bypass surgery

Anesthetic considerations for patients with MMD have been described in many literatures for both adult and pediatric populations [12–19]. Significant hemodynamic changes are expected throughout the perioperative period, and thus, it necessitates intensive care management. Hypertension and hypoventilation can potentially result in intracranial hemorrhage, likewise, intraoperative hypotension and hyperventilation can cause cerebral ischemia. The principles of safe anesthesia in neurosurgery, such as normotension, normocarbia, adequate oxygenation, normothermia, and normovolemia, are also applicable in revascularization surgery for patients with MMD. The anesthetic management of MMD presents unique challenges, as it can ensue further complications of the disease. Therefore, in-depth knowledge of pathophysiology and institutional guidelines for intraoperative optimal care of MMD patients improves perioperative care and long term outcomes [14, 17, 20]. Most of the following discussion highlights general anesthetic consideration in MMD (see **Table 3**).

Preoperative	• Evaluate cerebral ischemic risks, preexisting neurological deficits, stage of hemodynamic failure and adequacy of collateral circulation • Continue anti-seizure medication and perioperative anticoagulation/antiplatelet therapy decisions based on multidisciplinary team
Intraoperative	• Anesthetic goals: Maintenance of adequate cerebral perfusion and hemodynamic stability, ventilation to maintain normocarbia, and normothermia • Blood pressure goals: normotensive (Mean arterial pressue within 10–20% of preoperative baseline) and increase during temporary occlusion with vasopressors support (preferrable noradrenaline infusion) • Avoid dehydration, and target hematocrit around 35% • Adequate analgesia and scalp block (before mayfield pin placement) • Smooth emergence and avoid coughing on extubation • Balance ansethesia technique to facilitate immediate postoperative neurological assessment
Postoperative	• Patient admitted to intensive care unit for hemodynamic and neurological monitoring • Pain control with acetaminophen and postoperative sedation with fentanyl and dexmedetomidine also good choice • Ensure graft function and avoid hyperperfusion • Resume antiplatelet or anticoagulation

Table 3.
Perioperative considerations for revascularization surgery.

2.1 Preoperative anesthetic evaluation and premedication

Preoperative anesthetic assessment is paramount in reducing the complications associated with MMD and improving the surgical outcome. It must include detailed general medical, surgical history, physical exam, and assessment for signs and symptoms associated with MMD and coexisting comorbidities. Patients with MMD may have a significant preexisting neurologic deficit. Depending on the mode of presentation, hypertension can occur as a result of cerebral vascular incompetency. Inadequate treatment of hypertension may lead to perioperative cerebral infarction or stroke. History of frequent preoperative transient ischemic attacks indicates compromised cerebral collateral circulation and is a significant risk factor for perioperative complications [21–23]. Chronic cerebral ischemia may lead to neurologic deficits such as motor deficit, epilepsy, and mental retardation. MMD is linked to other medical conditions, including cardiovascular and renal systems, which have a direct impact on anesthetic management and postoperative outcomes. A multidisciplinary strategy is vital to improve the perioperative outcome and avoid complications, necessitating a high level of collaboration and communication with the surgeon. Suggested criteria in the selection of adult MMD patients for cerebral revascularization [17] (see **Table 4**). Thus, preoperative assessment allows early recognition of high-risk patients and reciprocal identification of the potential perioperative issues, and adequate preparation to deal with the challenges. In summary, the goal of preoperative anesthesia assessment involves recognizing risk factors for cerebral ischemia, pre-existing neurological deficits, degree of hemodynamic failure, adequacy of collateral circulation and vascular risk factors (diabetes, cardiovascular disease, hypertension), and optimize the patient's condition before surgery.

- Functional status: patient is able to perform activities of daily living (modified Rankin Scale>3)
- Neurological presentation: patient has recurrent (sensorymotor, speech, visual or gait disturbance) or progressive (crescendo focal deficit or global cognitive decline) neurological deficit(s) due to repeated TIAs, cerebral infarctions, cerebral hemorrhages or severe chronic hypoperfusion. The procedure is delayed for at least 6 weeks after the last cerebral infarction/haemorrhage
- Radiological features: the angiographic stage of the disease is Suzuki's stage II to IV
- Cerebral blood flow studies: dedicated imaging studies show at least significant hypoperfusion of the involve hemisphere or corresponding cortical area. The absence of cerebrovascular reactivity or the presence of a steal phenomenon is a stronger indicator of the severity of the disease, thus reinforcing the need for surgical intervention

Table 4.
Suggested criteria for revascularization surgery.

2.1.1 Preoperative investigation and imaging studies

Baseline preoperative laboratory investigation include a complete blood count, serum electrolytes, blood urea nitrogen, creatinine, glucose, and coagulation profile. An electrocardiogram (ECG), Echocardiogram, chest x-ray, and arterial blood gases may also be obtained. ECG abnormalities in MMD include ventricular enlargement and hypertrophy, ST-T wave changes, premature ventricular contraction, and right and left axis deviation [24–26]. A review of imaging studies especially cerebral angiography may help to identify the severity of the disease.

2.1.2 The Berlin moyamoya grading

It incorporated digital subtraction angiography, MRI, and cerebrovascular reserve capacity (CVRC) which allows to stratify clinical symptomatology and provides information on cerebrovascular function. Czabanka et al. propose the grading system which has three grades [27] (see **Table 5**).

2.1.3 Premedication

It is essential to review the chronic medical conditions of a patient with MMD. Review of medications is a vital part of anesthesia evaluation. Calcium channel

Variable	Characteristics	Points
DSA	Steno-occlusive lesion + Moyamoya vessels	1
	Steno-occlusive lesion+ moyamoya vessels +	2
	intracranial compensation routes	
	Steno-occlusive lesion+extra-intracranial compensation routs	3
MRI	No signs of ischemia/hemorrhage/atrophy	0
	Signs of ischemia/hemorrhage/atrophy	1
Cerebrovascular reserve capacity	No steal phenomenon (> – 5%)	0
	Steal phenomenon (<–5%)	2

Grades 1–2: mild; Grades 3–4: moderate; Grades 5–6: severe.

Table 5.
The Berlin grading system.

blockers and antiepileptic medications should be continued until the day of the surgery. Angiotensin-converting enzyme inhibitors (ACEi) and angiotensin receptor blockers should be stopped a day before surgery. Patients with symptomatic MMD and vaso-occlusive disease of the carotid and coronary artery, are usually on antiplatelet medications. Continuation of low dose aspirin in the perioperative period varies from center to center. In some centers, aspirin is continued until the day of the surgery whereas clopidogrel and other antiplatelet are discontinued five to seven days before surgery and bridged with low molecular weight heparin [9, 11]. Premedication with anxiolytics may be beneficial in pediatric patients, as crying causes hyperventilation that results in hypocarbia and hence, cerebral vasoconstriction and cerebral ischemia [18, 19]. Careful titration of anxiolytics is vital to reduce anxiety and on the other hand, to reduce the risk of cerebral vasodilation caused by hypoventilation and hypercarbia, as it may lead to raised intracranial pressure and cerebral hemorrhage. Adequate hydration during the preoperative period is deemed necessary to avoid compromised cerebral blood flow.

2.2 Intraoperative anesthesia consideration

2.2.1 Intraoperative monitoring technique

Intraoperative monitoring technique includes all routine basic physiological monitors also known as "Standard American Society of Anesthesiologists (ASA) monitors" such as Non-invasive blood pressure devices, Electrocardiography, Pulse oximetry for Oxygen saturation, capnography, and temperature monitoring. Additionally, an invasive intra-arterial catheter is inserted for continuous blood pressure monitoring preferably before induction to monitor and maintain the hemodynamics, central venous access, and Foley's catheter for urine output. Also, advanced cardiac output monitoring is usually considered in patients with significant cardiovascular and renal disease and to help in optimization of fluid status. However, there is limited data available on the usefulness of these cardiac output monitoring in intracranial bypass surgery. Likewise, cerebral function monitoring such as electroencephalogram (EEG) and somatosensory evoked potential (SSEP) have been used intraoperatively but less evidence available in the literature regarding their benefits [28–30]. Lastly, the role of other monitoring technique for global cerebral function such as transcranial Doppler, cerebral oximetry, and jugular bulb oxygen saturation have been reported; however, there is paucity of evidence available in the literature that their use help in early detection of cerebral ischemia or favorably impact the outcome [31–33].

2.2.2 Role of indocyanine green (ICG)

Indocyanine green video angiography (ICG-VA) is used in intracranial bypass surgery which is a non-invasive technique to assess the patency of a bypass graft or anastomosis [34–36]. ICG is a preservative-free powder (25 mg), which is diluted with 10 ml of distilled water (2.5 mg/ml). The technique requires intravenous injection of ICG and the direct application of a microscope with an integrated ICG camera on the operative field. The standard dose range from 5 to 25 mg. Intraoperative ICG-VA facilitates the identification of potential recipient vessels and detection of pathological flow patterns [35]. The main disadvantage of ICG angiogram is the failure to visualize deeper vasculatures. ICG injection may cause erroneous readings on the pulse oximeter and can cause anaphylactic reactions [37, 38].

2.2.3 Choice of anesthesia techniques

General anesthesia is recommended for revascularization surgery. The goal of anesthesia induction is to maintain hemodynamics, oxygenation, and ventilation. It also aims to avoid a decrease in cerebral perfusion pressure (CPP) and increased intracranial pressure (ICP), which are attributed to anesthetic drugs and airway maneuvers. The choice of induction technique for general anesthesia (intravenous versus inhalational agents) has been debated and depends on patient factors (pediatric versus adult), surgical factors (use of neurophysiologic monitoring), and potential for compromised or difficult airway [18, 39, 40]. Sakamoto et al. investigated the perioperative course of 216 patients undergoing revascularization; they concluded that the incidence of postoperative ischemic events was associated with the severity of the disease and surgical procedure than with other factors, including anesthetic management (inhaled, IV, and balanced anesthesia) [40].

Sato et al. studied the effect of total intravenous anesthesia (TIVA) versus volatile anesthetic on cerebral circulation in MMD and concluded that volatile agents might reduce the regional cortical blood flow and hence, inducing intracerebral steal; this was not observed with TIVA [41]. More recently, studies demonstrated improved outcomes when TIVA is used [42], whereas other studies have not shown a significant difference between TIVA versus inhalational agents in MMD [43]. Many centers are routinely utilizing total intravenous anesthesia (TIVA) with target-controlled infusion (TCI) of propofol and opioids (remifentanil) for the neurosurgical procedure [44]. In TCI, the infusion pumps are set to deliver a bolus on induction followed by a maintenance infusion based on the patient's demographics. TIVA with propofol and remifentanil offers theoretical advantages for neurosurgical procedures such as careful and easy titration of anesthetic to maintain the hemodynamics intraoperatively; and most notably rapid, smooth emergence with early recovery of neur0cognitive function without postoperative nausea and vomiting. Additionally, TIVA is an anesthetic of choice in neurosurgery during neurophysiological monitoring (SSEP). In conclusion, more prospective studies are needed to determine the influence of different anesthetic techniques on revascularization surgery and its outcome.

2.2.4 Oxygenation and ventilation strategies

Cerebral oxygenation depends on the content of oxygen in the arterial blood, cerebral blood flow, and metabolic activity of brain tissue. All of these elements can be altered in patients with chronic cerebral ischemia. Intraoperative goals of oxygenation and ventilation should be maintaining normo-oxygenation and normocarbia [18, 19, 45]. Carbon dioxide is a potent modulator of cerebrovascular tone and influences the cerebral blood flow with changes in ventilation and can be a potential factor in determining neurologic complications perioperatively. In one systematic review, cerebrovascular reactivity to PaCO2 is maintained under both propofol and inhalational agents provided anesthetic concentration within the range used in clinical anesthesia [46]. Sumikawa et al., intraoperative hypocapnia (PaCo2 30-35 mm Hg) is linked to delayed recovery of consciousness and postoperative neurologic deficits [47]. Therefore, one should aim at maintaining normocarbia with PaCO2 between 35 to 40 mm Hg.

2.2.5 Hemodynamic management

Effective and prompt hemodynamic control is crucial during the perioperative period. Both hypotension and hypertension have a detrimental effect on postoperative outcomes. Hypotension is poorly tolerated by patients with MMD and leads to cerebral ischemia and thrombosis of the bypass graft postoperatively. Likewise, hypertension results in intracranial hemorrhage especially at the site of anastomosis either during or after the surgery. The incidence and extent of postoperative cerebral ischemia can be decreased by adopting individualized perioperative blood pressure management [48]. The optimal blood pressure target during surgery is not well described but the general recommendation is to keep the blood pressure within 10% to 20% of the preoperative baseline blood pressure for all patients [18, 19, 45]. Careful titration of anesthetic during induction and maintenance of anesthesia is critical in regulating the blood pressure. Any episode of hypotension (systolic less than 100 mm Hg) should be treated promptly with vasoactive drugs. Similarly, persistent perioperative hypertension should be controlled with drugs such as hydralazine, esmolol, or labetalol.

2.2.6 Fluid and blood products

The goal of fluid management is to maintain normovolemia and a hematocrit between 30 and 35% [49]. Hemodilution and polycythemia both carry the risk of perioperative cerebral ischemia [50]. So, careful titration and control of blood viscosity are vital; this is accomplished by replacing insensible losses, blood loss, and urine output with a combination of normal saline and 5% albumin or blood products. Though some studies have recommended a hypervolemia state to avoid the issues associated with hypotension and decreased cerebral perfusion [51]. Arterial blood gas, electrolyte, glucose, and hematocrit should be measured at regular intervals throughout the case with the target of maintaining normal values. It has been suggested that hematocrit of about 30–35% balances the oxygen blood content and blood viscosity and promotes sufficient oxygen delivery extrapolated from the cardiac surgery. Advanced cardiac output monitoring is utilized in assessing volume status, fluid responsiveness, and guiding fluid therapy, and the need for vasopressors.

2.2.7 Temperature management

Normothermia is commonly advocated in neurosurgery to avoid post-operative shivering, surgical site infection, cardiac arrhythmia, acidosis, and coagulopathy. Mild hypothermia is considered as it offers some degree of neuroprotection against cerebral hypoxia and ischemia by reducing the cerebral metabolic rate. However, there have been few studies and no randomized clinical trials conducted. Moreover, the role of cerebral-protective techniques such as inducing burst suppression with the administration of propofol or barbiturates or hypothermia at the time of temporary artery clamping, is debatable and is dependent on the centers and surgeons' preferences.

2.2.8 Analgesia

The importance of perioperative control of pain in MMD cannot be overstated. Pain is associated with neuroendocrine responses, resulting in an increase in cerebral metabolism that is detrimental to MMD. A postoperative cerebral infarction may be associated with inadequate pain control. Therefore, adequate perioperative analgesia may reduce the risk of cerebral ischemia or infarction [40]. Multimodal analgesia (MMA) strategy is often employed to optimize pain control and limit the undesired side effect simultaneously. MMA includes the use of opioids coupled with acetaminophen, gabapentin, or pregabalin, and non-narcotic analgesics such as tramadol and COX-2 inhibitors [52, 53]. The use of local anesthetic and regional anesthesia is also recommended. Patient-controlled analgesia can also be considered in the postoperative period.

2.2.9 Regional anesthesia

Regional anesthesia offers perioperative analgesia and facilitates smooth emergence. Harvey, Cushing, and George Crile, first described the role of local anesthetic infiltration or regional anesthetics of the scalp for craniotomies in the early 1900s [54]. Girvin et al. first described the scalp nerve block technique in 1986 for use during awake craniotomy. It comprises of blocking six nerves that provide the sensory innervation of the scalp, on either side of the scalp, with infiltration of local anesthetics (2-3 ml) for each nerve. These nerves consist of the supraorbital, supratrochlear, zygomaticotemporal, auriculotemporal, lesser occipital, and greater occipital nerves, usually given bilaterally. Scalp block effectively blunts the hemodynamic response preoperatively. Also, scalp block has been proven to be superior over a sham group (with saline) in terms of hemodynamic stability and decreased anesthetic requirement during cranial fixation [55, 56]. Scalp block's effect also extends into the postoperative period and has proved to decrease the incidence and severity of postoperative pain [57]. In summary, the incorporation of regional anesthesia has led to a smooth intraoperative course and improved postoperative patient comfort.

2.3 Emergence and extubation

The aim of emergence from anesthesia includes smooth, rapid emergence and extubation; also avoidance of straining, bucking, and coughing, and complete, pain-free awakening. Use of lidocaine intra-tracheal before extubation will safeguard against coughing and bucking and repeat scalp block at the end of surgery. A smooth emergence with controlled hemodynamics is vital to prevent hemorrhagic complications and graft thrombosis. The tenuous cerebral blood supply places patients with MMD at increased risk of perioperative morbidity during revascularization procedures because of the hemodynamic changes that may occur throughout induction, maintenance, and emergence. The consensus is to maintain CPP at or above the baseline perioperatively. The principle of neuroanesthesia care such as normotension, normovolemia, norm0-oxygenation, normocapnia, and normothermia; must be implemented during the emergence and post-extubation period.

2.4 Postoperative intensive care

Postoperative care of MMD patients undergoing revascularization surgery preferably takes place in the intensive care unit. They need to be closely monitored for any hemodynamic and neurological changes, as postoperative ischemic events have been attributed to hemodynamic swings. Invasive monitoring to continue throughout the journey to the ICU. It is crucial to avoid both hypotension and hypertension that may cause graft thrombosis and bleed respectively. Optimal control of blood pressure, oxygen supply, ventilation may help to prevent the incidence of perioperative cerebral ischemic events.

Intravenous fluid administration to maintain normovolemia and starting aspirin on the first postoperative day has been recommended. Adequate analgesia is provided to prevent agitation and increased stress, which may affect the bypass. Postoperative sedation/analgesia with dexmedetomidine and fentanyl infusion is a good choice.

3. Postoperative neurological complications and outcome

Multiple risk factors have been implicated with perioperative complications in MMD patients, such as patient comorbidities, the severity of the disease, type of surgery, type of revascularization procedure, and nonsurgical hemodynamic risk factors.

3.1 Cerebral ischemia

The incidence of postoperative cerebral ischemia has been reported to be approximately 3.5% in adult patients and 16.9% in pediatric patients [32, 58]. Sakamoto et al. studied the risk factors for perioperative complications in revascularization surgery and found that the severity of the disease, history of TIA, and indirect bypass procedures were the major determinants for postoperative neurological deficits [59]. Similarly, Zhao et al. recently found that advanced Suzuki stage and preoperative ischemic presentation were independent risk factors for postoperative ischemia [60]. Lastly, The Carotid Occlusion Surgery Study (COSS) investigators found that the mechanism of stroke was usually attributed to hypoperfusion and the occurrence of artery-to-artery emboli or thrombosis [61].

3.2 Cerebral hyperfusion syndrome (CHS)

CHS was first reported by Uno et al. in a patient with MMD after extracranial-intracranial bypass in 1998 [62]. Since 1998, CHS has been reported in both pediatric and adult MMD patients after direct revascularization surgery.

The incidence of cerebral hyperperfusion in patients with occlusive cerebrovascular disease is reported at 17% after bypass surgeries, and 0.4% to 20% after carotid endarterectomy [63]. In another study, the incidence of CHS in MMD patients after direct surgical revascularization was reported to be 21.5% [64]. Adult-onset, hemorrhagic presentation, and increased preoperative cerebral blood volume were the risk factors for developing CHS [63]. The most common symptoms are transient neurological deficits, followed by hemorrhage and seizure [65]. CHS after surgical revascularization is caused by an increase in the cerebral blood flow, control of blood pressure postoperatively is the direct way to prevent or treat CHS. Active treatment of CHS should be considered in a patient with postoperative neurologic deficits such as headache, seizure, or transient focal neurological deficits. The strict control of blood pressure at targets less than 120/80 mm Hg, and routine postoperative monitoring of cerebral blood flow using transcranial Doppler and dynamic imaging techniques (computerized tomography or magnetic resonance perfusion) to be effective in preventing permanent neurological sequelae secondary to cerebral hyperperfusion syndrome [63, 66].

4. Special anesthetic consideration in MMD

4.1 Anesthetic consideration in the obstetric patient with MMD

Parturients with moyamoya syndrome should be treated with tight blood pressure control. Hypotension and hypertension should be avoided. Peripartum pain control is crucial to preventing pain-related hyperventilation and resultant cerebral vasoconstriction. Because cerebral aneurysms may develop with disease progression, these patients are at higher risk of intracranial hemorrhage than the general population. The development of cerebral aneurysms may be secondary to chronic hypertension or regional vessel constriction in moyamoya. Additionally, multiple tiny collateral arterioles develop at sites of proximal arterial occlusion which are prone to rupture. Hypercoagulability, venous stasis, and endothelial lesion are common in pregnancy and may contribute to stroke. Therefore, the anesthetic goals for a parturient with known Moyamoya syndrome are to avoid hypertension, which can precipitate the hemorrhage, and avoid hypotension or hypocapnia that can reduce placental perfusion and the already compromised cerebral blood flow. The decision for timing and method of delivery in MMD patients is based on reducing risks associated with hemodynamic instability. Control of hemodynamic fluctuations, minimizing anxiety and pain, and Valsalva, and meticulous fluid management during intrapartum are the main components for maintaining optimal end-organ perfusion of the mother and fetus. More than 70% of parturients with MMD undergo an elective cesarean section. This is the delivery route of choice to prevent intracranial hemorrhage due to hypertension during labor. General anesthesia and neuraxial anesthesia have been reported as successful for the cesarean section [67–71]. However, both techniques are associated with sudden hypotension which may progress to ischemic events. General anesthesia is chosen for better control of hypotension (common in spinal anesthesia, leading to cerebral hypoperfusion). Tracheal intubation during general anesthesia may cause hypertension resulting in intracranial hemorrhage and general anesthesia also carries the risk of aspiration. Care should be taken during direct laryngoscopy to reduce sympathetic drive. Also, the technique could prevent hyperventilation secondary to maternal anxiety, which causes hypocapnia and decreases cerebral blood flow. Normotension and normocapnia should be the goals during general anesthesia. Vaginal delivery is considered in MMD patients at low risk for intracranial hemorrhage, such as those who underwent bypass surgery or without a history of bleeding [72]. Most affected parturient undergo successful cesarean deliveries under neuraxial anesthesia (spinal, epidural, or combined spinal-epidural anesthesia), often with invasive arterial hemodynamic monitoring; as it provides easier monitoring for neurological changes as well as preventing hypertension associated with intubation during general anesthesia. Additionally, a multidisciplinary approach (i.e., anesthesiologist, obstetrician, fetal medicine, and neurosurgery) is necessary to constantly manage underlying diseases.

4.2 Anesthetic consideration in a pediatric patient with MMD

Pediatric patients with MMD have a higher baseline cerebral metabolic rate of oxygen consumption and thus poorly tolerate any reduction in cerebral blood flow. Therefore, these children should be maintained with a normal or higher than normal mean arterial pressure; normocapnia to prevent hypocapnia mediated cerebral vasoconstriction and also prevent hypercapnia leading to cerebral blood flow steal phenomenon; adequate hydration; analgesia; and normothermia [15].

Pre-operatively children have undergone workup for neurological symptoms such as cerebral vascular imaging (MRI or MRA) and are typically on anti-platelet or anti-seizure medications. Additionally, these children are on medication (such as midodrine) that keeps the blood pressure up as these stenotic cerebral arteries depend on high blood pressure, and any medication that decreases the blood pressure can be detrimental. Children are usually anxious from possible parental separation; may benefit from the use of pre-anesthesia anxiolysis as well as the comforting presence of the parent in the operating room or virtual reality (music etc). Crying can lead to hyperventilation and hypocapnia. Additionally, these patients must be kept well hydrated to allow for adequate blood volume in the context of anesthesia-induced vasodilation. Since these patients are nil-per-oral, they should be given intravenous fluids of around one and half times their maintenance requirements pre-operatively. Also, a thorough history and physical examination necessary to determine any other associated conditions such as sickle cell disease, neurofibromatosis type 1, and trisomy 21.

Intra-operatively, these children may be induced intravenously if they have an intravenous line in place or by inhalation. Outcomes for induction are similar for both these approaches provided the blood pressure and ventilation is maintained.

Intravenous maintenance with combined propofol and remifentanil may be better compared to inhalational maintenance as studies have shown reduced cerebral oxygenation with inhalational agents perhaps due to the cerebral steal phenomenon [42, 43, 73]. Phenylephrine infusion is utilized to maintain the mean arterial pressure. Hyperventilation and hypoventilation must be avoided as they are associated with negative outcomes. Sympathetic response to laryngoscopy and intubation must be blunted with intravenous lidocaine, opioid, or short-acting beta-blockers. To maintain blood pressure and ventilation, it is essential to monitor these patients with an invasive arterial line, pulse oximetry, capnography, ECG, and temperature. Additionally, intra-operative EEG is recommended. A urine catheter to monitor urine output with careful monitoring of fluid balance is needed to maintain normovolemia. Central venous access is rarely required but can be utilized in patients with difficult intravenous access. Intravenous fluids must not contain glucose.

Post-operatively, smooth extubation with adequate analgesia, hydration, and normothermia is necessary as not to potentially jeopardize cerebral blood flow. Patients who have undergone indirect revascularization are still at risk of post-operative stroke. Analgesia must be maintained usually with an opioid-based patient-controlled technique supplemented with other analgesics such as acetaminophen. Anti-emetics must be given to prevent nausea or vomiting. Recovery must be ideally carried out by trained pediatric intensive care nurses experienced in managing Moyamoya disease. Transfer of care to a high dependency unit is recommended after recovery.

4.3 Anesthetic consideration for MMD patients going for non-revascularization surgery

4.3.1 Laparoscopic surgery

Laparoscopic surgery has gained tremendous popularity in recent years. The key element in laparoscopic surgery is the creation of pneumoperitoneum with carbon dioxide insufflation. The physiological changes especially cardiopulmonary alterations during laparoscopic surgery occur mainly due to the creation of pneumoperitoneum and positioning of the patient. Similarly, cerebral hemodynamic changes (including changes in cerebral perfusion and intracranial pressure) also occur during the creation of pneumoperitoneum and positioning of the patient. Anesthesia goals for MMD patients undergoing laparoscopic surgery are to allow physiological changes during surgery with minimal effects on the body's vital organs and rapid and smooth recovery. Induction of anesthesia should be carried out with careful titration of anesthetic drugs to avoid hemodynamic fluctuations. Airway manipulation should be minimized to avoid sympathetic surge. Nakanishi et al. used Laryngeal mask airway ProSeal successfully in a MMD patient who underwent laparoscopic cholecystectomy [74]. The author proposes the use of LMA ProSeal as an effective alternative with minimal hemodynamic change, compared with tracheal intubation [75]. Moreover, Lee et al. reported a case of intracranial hemorrhage during laparoscopic cholecystectomy due to unrecognized MMD [76]. Hence, rigorous ventilatory management utilizing End-tidal CO2 and arterial CO2 during pneumoperitoneum and arterial blood pressure for continuous monitoring of hemodynamic changes is mandatory. The intraoperative aim is to maintain blood pressure, oxygen saturation, ventilation, and smooth emergence from anesthesia.

4.3.2 Cardiac surgery

Patients with MMD undergoing cardiac surgery requiring cardiopulmonary bypass (CPB) pose considerable anesthetic challenges. CPB is a technique in which a machine temporarily takes over the function of the heart and lung.

CPB in moyamoya patients has a high risk of decreasing cerebral perfusion pressure due to the perfusion pressure variability in the initial stages of CPB and non-pulsatile flow. Moreover, the risk of hypocapnic cerebral vasoconstriction and hypercapnic cerebral steal is a well-recognized phenomenon. Preserving the autoregulation of the cerebral blood flow is key to prevent cerebral ischemia. Case report proposes the use of an Intra-aortic balloon pump (IABP) that produces pulsatile flow which facilitates maintaining a higher perfusion pressure (mean arterial pressure > 80 mm Hg) and reduces the vasoconstrictors' requirement [77–79]. Regional cerebral oxygen saturation (rSO2) monitoring for cerebral blood flow; is a useful tool and provides real-time cerebral blood flow; the goal is to keep cerebral saturation at 80% of the baseline value. The key strategy is to keep the blood pressure, PaCO2, hematocrit, and body temperature to normal and should be adjusted rigorously intraoperatively. Off-pump coronary artery bypass (OPCAB) is a safe procedure that avoids the risk of CPB related hypotensive brain ischemia, for multi-vessel coronary patients with moyamoya disease [80, 81].

5. Conclusion

Moyamoya disease (MMD) is a unique, slowly progressive cerebral vasculopathy with an incidence of 0.09–10/100,000 individuals. It is highly prevalent in East Asia. It has an unknown etiology and classically presents with symptoms of headaches, transient ischemic attacks such as dysarthria, hemiparesis, cognitive decline, aphasia, and seizures. Early diagnosis and early treatment are effective in preventing further deterioration. Medical treatment is aimed at managing symptoms and typically includes anti-seizure, antihypertensive, and antiplatelet therapy. Surgical revascularization is the cornerstone in treating MMD patients to reduce further ischemic insults and neurological deterioration. Its unique pathophysiology requires anesthesiologists to strategize an individualized anesthetic plan and close-in line communications with the neurosurgical team. Premedication is essential in pediatric patients undergoing revascularization surgery as the goal is to avoid crying and hyperventilation which provokes cerebral vasoconstriction. Perioperative management of moyamoya disease has a direct influence on the outcomes of the surgery. The key goals of perioperative management are maintenance of normotension, normovolaemia, normocapnia and normothermia, and adequate analgesia. Postoperatively, patients are admitted to the intensive care unit for close hemodynamic assessment and timely neurological assessment. Effective analgesia and fluid resuscitation must be employed postoperatively. Antiepileptic drugs are continued perioperatively, and antiplatelet agents are started postoperatively.

Acknowledgements

We would like to acknowledge the contribution of Ms. Nadia Ibrahim for her editorial help.

Conflict of interest

The authors declare no conflict of interest.

Notes

The authors searched all published literatures on Moyamoya disease from Medical Literature Analysis and Retrieval System Online database (MEDLINE via Pubmed) and Google Scholar database and the Excerpta Medica database (EMBASE). Also, the authors used the following search keywords in combination with "Moyamoya disease, Anesthesia, Diagnosis, Medical Management, Surgical management, Revascularization surgery, Perioperative management, Postoperative complication, Pediatric anesthesia, Obstetric anesthesia, Laparoscopic surgery, Cardiac surgery.

Author details

Muhammad Jaffar Khan*, Jazib Hassan, Sumayya Aboobacker, Tarek Tageldin, Jafar Faraj and Mohamed El-Arref
Department of Anesthesia, Perioperative Medicine and Critical Care, Hamad Medical Corporation, Doha, Qatar

*Address all correspondence to: jafar06khan@gmail

References

[1] Kuroda S, Houkin K. Moyamoya disease: current concepts and future perspectives. Vol. 7, The Lancet Neurology. Elsevier; 2008. p. 1056-66.

[2] Scott RM, Smith ER. Moyamoya Disease and Moyamoya Syndrome. N Engl J Med [Internet]. 2009 Mar 19 [cited 2021 Jan 30];360(12):1226-37. Available from: https://www.nejm.org/doi/10.1056/NEJMra0804622

[3] Yamani M, Obaid EF, Hemida AH. Moyamoya Syndrome in a 32-Year-Old Male With Sickle Cell Anemia. Cureus. 2020 Aug 25;

[4] Zhang H, Zheng L, Feng L. Epidemiology, diagnosis and treatment of moyamoya disease (Review). Exp Ther Med [Internet]. 2019 Jan 25 [cited 2021 Feb 6];17(3):1977-84. Available from: http://www.spandidos-publications.com/10.3892/etm.2019.7198/abstract

[5] Gupta A, Tyagi A, Romo M, Amoroso KC, Sonia F. Moyamoya Disease: A Review of Current Literature. Cureus. 2020 Aug 31;

[6] Liao X, Deng J, Dai W, Zhang T, Yan J. Rare variants of RNF213 and moyamoya/non-moyamoya intracranial artery stenosis/occlusion disease risk: A meta-analysis and systematic review. Environ Health Prev Med [Internet]. 2017 Nov 2 [cited 2021 Feb 6];22(1):75. Available from: http://environhealthprevmed.biomedcentral.com/articles/10.1186/s12199-017-0680-1

[7] Willis RC on the P and T of SO of the C of, Diseases HLSRG for R on M for I. Guidelines for Diagnosis and Treatment of Moyamoya Disease (Spontaneous Occlusion of the Circle of Willis): Esearch Committee on the Pathology and Treatment of Spontaneous Occlusion of the Circle of Willis; Health Labour Sciences Research Grant for Resear. Neurol Med Chir (Tokyo) [Internet]. 2012 [cited 2021 Jan 29];52(5):245-66. Available from: http://jlc.jst.go.jp/DN/JST.JSTAGE/nmc/52.245?lang=en&from=CrossRef&type=abstract

[8] Suzuki J, Takaku A. Cerebrovascular "Moyamoya#x201D; Disease: Disease Showing Abnormal Net-Like Vessels in Base of Brain. Arch Neurol [Internet]. 1969 Mar 1 [cited 2021 Jan 29];20(3):288-99. Available from: https://jamanetwork.com/journals/jamaneurology/fullarticle/568758

[9] Uchiyama S, Yamazaki M, Ishikawa T, Yamaguchi K, Kawamata T. Diagnosis and Management of Moyamoya Disease. Case Rep Neurol [Internet]. 2020 Dec 14 [cited 2021 Feb 6];12(Suppl1):137-42. Available from: https://www.karger.com/Article/FullText/505967

[10] Liu JJ, Steinberg GK. Direct Versus Indirect Bypass for Moyamoya Disease. Vol. 28, Neurosurgery Clinics of North America. W.B. Saunders; 2017. p. 361-374.

[11] Acker G, Fekonja L, Vajkoczy P. Surgical management of moyamoya disease [Internet]. Vol. 49, Stroke. Lippincott Williams and Wilkins; 2018 [cited 2021 Feb 6]. p. 476-82. Available from: http://stroke.ahajournals.org

[12] Varghes MP, Kuzhiyelil KR, Lionel KR, Singh G, Mariappan R. Anesthetic Management of Encephalo-duroarteriosynangiosis (EDAS) for Moyamoya Disease: A Retrospective Study. In: Abstracts of 21st Annual Conference of the Indian Society of Neuroanaesthesiology and Critical Care (ISNACC 2020) [Internet]. Thieme Medical and Scientific Publishers Private Ltd.; 2020 [cited 2021 Feb 6]. p. A003. Available from: http://www.thieme-connect.de/DOI/DOI?10.1055/s-0040-1709570

[13] Li C, Zhang N, Yu S, Xu Y, Yao Y, Zeng M, et al. Individualized

Perioperative Blood Pressure Management for Adult Moyamoya Disease: Experience from 186 Consecutive Procedures. J Stroke Cerebrovasc Dis. 2021 Jan 1;30(1):105413.

[14] Williams GW, Jones WS, Chaudhry R, Cai C, Pednekar GS, Long AC, et al. Intraoperative Anesthesiology Management and Patient Outcomes for Surgical Revascularization for Moyamoya Disease: A Review and Clinical Experience. J Neurol Surgery, Part A Cent Eur Neurosurg [Internet]. 2019 [cited 2021 Feb 6];80(3):143-8. Available from: https://pubmed.ncbi.nlm.nih.gov/30818408/

[15] Giustini AJ, Stone SA, Ramamoorthy C. Moyamoya disease in children and its anesthetic implications: A review [Internet]. Vol. 30, Paediatric Anaesthesia. Blackwell Publishing Ltd; 2020 [cited 2021 Feb 1]. p. 1191-8. Available from: https://onlinelibrary.wiley.com/doi/10.1111/pan.14001

[16] Williams GW, Jones WS, Chaudhry R, Cai C, Pednekar GS, Long AC, et al. Intraoperative Anesthesiology Management and Patient Outcomes for Surgical Revascularization for Moyamoya Disease: A Review and Clinical Experience. J Neurol Surgery, Part A Cent Eur Neurosurg [Internet]. 2019 May 28 [cited 2021 Jan 30];80(3):143-8. Available from: http://www.thieme-connect.de/DOI/DOI?10.1055/s-0039-1677823

[17] WW G. Effect of Intraoperative Anesthetic Management on Patient Outcomes for Surgical Revascularization for Moyamoya Disease: A 7-year Retrospective Study. J Anesth Intensive Care Med. 2017;3(4).

[18] Chui J, Manninen P, Sacho RH, Venkatraghavan L. Anesthetic management of patients undergoing intracranial bypass procedures [Internet]. Vol. 120, Anesthesia and Analgesia. Lippincott Williams and Wilkins; 2015 [cited 2021 Jan 30]. p. 193-203. Available from: http://journals.lww.com/00000539-201501000-00027

[19] Parray T, Martin TW, Siddiqui S. Moyamoya disease: A review of the disease and anesthetic management [Internet]. Vol. 23, Journal of Neurosurgical Anesthesiology. 2011 [cited 2021 Jan 30]. p. 100-9. Available from: https://journals.lww.com/00008506-201104000-00003

[20] Ha EJ, Kim KH, Wang KC, Phi JH, Lee JY, Choi JW, et al. Long-Term Outcomes of Indirect Bypass for 629 Children With Moyamoya Disease: Longitudinal and Cross-Sectional Analysis. Stroke [Internet]. 2019 Nov 1 [cited 2021 Feb 1];50(11):3177-83. Available from: https://www.ahajournals.org/doi/10.1161/STROKEAHA.119.025609

[21] Zhai X, Mao L, Wang H, Zhang X, Hang C, Wu W, et al. Risk Factors Associated with Neurologic Deterioration After Combined Direct and Indirect Revascularization in Patients with Moyamoya Disease on the East Coast of China. World Neurosurg. 2018 Oct 1;118:e92–e98.

[22] Qian Y, Huang B, Hu Z, Wang J, Zhao P, Li X. Analysis of Factors Related to Cerebral Infarction after Direct Bypass Surgery in Adults with Moyamoya Disease. Cerebrovasc Dis [Internet]. 2020 Mar 1 [cited 2021 Feb 6];49(1):55-61. Available from: https://www.karger.com/Article/FullText/504743

[23] Park W, Ahn JS, Lee HS, Park JC, Kwun BD. Risk Factors for Newly Developed Cerebral Infarction after Surgical Revascularization for Adults with Moyamoya Disease. World Neurosurg. 2016 Aug 1;92:65-73.

[24] Nam TM, Jo K Il, Yeon JY, Hong SC, Kim JS. Coronary heart disease in moyamoya disease: Are they concomitant or coincidence? J

Korean Med Sci [Internet]. 2015 Apr 1 [cited 2021 Jan 19];30(4):470-4. Available from: https://jkms.org/DOIx.php?id=10.3346/jkms.2015.30.4.470

[25] Larson AS, Savastano L, Klaas J, Lanzino G. Cardiac manifestations in a western moyamoya disease population: a single-center descriptive study and review. Neurosurg Rev [Internet]. 2020 Jun 7 [cited 2021 Jan 19];1-8. Available from: https://link.springer.com/article/10.1007/s10143-020-01327-x

[26] Lee JH, Youn TJ, Yoon YE, Park JJ, Hong SJ, Chun EJ, et al. Coronary artery stenosis in moyamoya disease: Tissue characterization by 256-slice multi-detector CT and virtual histology [Internet]. Vol. 127, Circulation. Lippincott Williams & Wilkins Hagerstown, MD; 2013 [cited 2021 Jan 19]. p. 2063-5. Available from: https://www.ahajournals.org/doi/10.1161/CIRCULATIONAHA.112.136473

[27] Czabanka M, Peña-Tapia P, Schubert GA, Heppner FL, Martus P, Horn P, et al. Proposal for a new grading of Moyamoya disease in adult patients. Cerebrovasc Dis [Internet]. 2011 Jul [cited 2021 Feb 1];32(1):41-50. Available from: https://www.karger.com/Article/FullText/326077

[28] Wong DHW, McLeod DH. Intraoperative monitoring in patients with Moyamoya disease [Internet]. Vol. 42, Canadian Journal of Anaesthesia. Springer; 1995 [cited 2021 Jan 20]. p. 1064-5. Available from: https://link.springer.com/article/10.1007/BF03011087

[29] Vendrame M, Kaleyias J, Loddenkemper T, Smith E, McClain C, Rockoff M, et al. Electroencephalogram monitoring during intracranial surgery for moyamoya disease. Pediatr Neurol [Internet]. 2011 Jun 1 [cited 2021 Jan 20];44(6):427-32. Available from: http://www.pedneur.com/article/S0887899411000464/fulltext

[30] López JR. Neurophysiologic intraoperative monitoring of pediatric cerebrovascular surgery [Internet]. Vol. 26, Journal of Clinical Neurophysiology. 2009 [cited 2021 Jan 20]. p. 85-94. Available from: http://journals.lww.com/00004691-200904000-00006

[31] Oshima H, Katayama Y, Hirayama T, Koshinaga M, Yamamoto T. Intra-operative monitoring of jugular bulb oxygen saturation in patients with Moyamoya disease. In: Clinical Neurology and Neurosurgery [Internet]. Elsevier B.V.; 1997 [cited 2021 Jan 20]. Available from: https://pubmed.ncbi.nlm.nih.gov/9409417/

[32] Oshima H, Katayama Y, Hirayama T. Intracerebral steal phenomenon associated with global hyperemia in moyamoya disease during revascularization surgery. J Neurosurg [Internet]. 2000 [cited 2021 Jan 20];92(6):949-54. Available from: https://pubmed.ncbi.nlm.nih.gov/10839254/

[33] Murata Y, Katayama Y, Sakatani K, Fukaya C, Kano T. Evaluation of extracranial-intracranial arterial bypass function by using near-infrared spectroscopy. J Neurosurg [Internet]. 2003 Aug 1 [cited 2021 Jan 20];99(2):304-10. Available from: https://thejns.org/view/journals/j-neurosurg/99/2/article-p304.xml

[34] Tanabe N, Yamamoto S, Kashiwazaki D, Akioka N, Kuwayama N, Noguchi K, et al. Indocyanine green visualization of middle meningeal artery before craniotomy during surgical revascularization for moyamoya disease. Acta Neurochir (Wien) [Internet]. 2017 Mar 1 [cited 2021 Feb 6];159(3):567-75. Available from: https://link.springer.com/article/10.1007/s00701-016-3060-5

[35] Goldberg J, Vajkoczy P, Hecht N. Indocyanine green videoangiography for recipient vessel stratification in superficial temporal artery–middle

cerebral artery bypass surgery. J Neurosurg [Internet]. 2020 Aug 28 [cited 2021 Feb 6];1(aop):1-9. Available from: https://thejns.org/view/journals/j-neurosurg/aop/article-10.3171-2020.5.JNS20642/article-10.3171-2020.5.JNS20642.xml

[36] Dodier P, Auzinger T, Mistelbauer G, Wang W Te, Ferraz-Leite H, Gruber A, et al. Novel Software-Derived Workflow in Extracranial–Intracranial Bypass Surgery Validated by Transdural Indocyanine Green Videoangiography. In: World Neurosurgery. Elsevier Inc.; 2020. p. e892-902.

[37] Matsuzaki M, Ishii K, Nishida A, Motozawa N, Fujimori M, Hamada M, et al. Artifactual reduction in oxygen saturation readings affected by indocyanine green in ophthalmic angiography. Jpn J Ophthalmol [Internet]. 2020 Sep 1 [cited 2021 Feb 6];64(5):516-23. Available from: https://link.springer.com/article/10.1007/s10384-020-00760-1

[38] Kim M, Lee S, Park JC, Jang DM, Ha S Il, Kim JU, et al. Anaphylactic Shock After Indocyanine Green Video Angiography During Cerebrovascular Surgery. World Neurosurg. 2020 Jan 1;133:74-79.

[39] Jagdevan S, Sriganesh K, Pandey P, Reddy M, Rao GSU. Anesthetic factors and outcome in children undergoing indirect revascularization procedure for moyamoya disease: An Indian perspective [Internet]. Vol. 63, Neurology India. Medknow Publications; 2015 [cited 2021 Jan 20]. p. 702-6. Available from: http://www.neurologyindia.com/text.asp?2015/63/5/702/166575

[40] Sakamoto T, Kawaguchi M, Kurehara K, Kitaguchi K, Furuya H, Karasawa J. Risk factors for neurologic deterioration after revascularization surgery in patients with moyamoya disease. Anesth Analg [Internet]. 1997 Nov [cited 2021 Jan 20];85(5):1060-5. Available from: http://journals.lww.com/00000539-199711000-00018

[41] Sato K, Shirane R, Kato M, Yoshimoto T. Effect of inhalational anesthesia on cerebral circulation in Moyamoya disease. J Neurosurg Anesthesiol [Internet]. 1999 Jan [cited 2021 Jan 20];11(1):25-30. Available from: http://journals.lww.com/00008506-199901000-00005

[42] Adachi K, Yamamoto Y, Kameyama E, Suzuki H, Horinouchi T. Early postoperative complications in patients with moyamoya disease: A comparison of inhaled anesthesia with total intravenous anesthesia (TIVA). Japanese J Anesthesiol [Internet]. 2005 Jun 1 [cited 2021 Jan 20];54(6):653-7. Available from: https://europepmc.org/article/med/15966384

[43] Kikuta K ichiro, Takagi Y, Nozaki K, Yamada K, Miyamoto S, Kataoka H, et al. Effects of intravenous anesthesia with propofol on regional cortical blood flow and intracranial pressure in surgery for moyamoya disease. Surg Neurol. 2007 Oct 1;68(4):421-424.

[44] Preethi J, Bidkar PU, Cherian A, Dey A, Srinivasan S, Adinarayanan S, et al. Comparison of total intravenous anesthesia vs. inhalational anesthesia on brain relaxation, intracranial pressure, and hemodynamics in patients with acute subdural hematoma undergoing emergency craniotomy: a randomized control trial. Eur J Trauma Emerg Surg [Internet]. 2019 Oct 29 [cited 2021 Feb 6];1-7. Available from: https://link.springer.com/article/10.1007/s00068-019-01249-4

[45] Wanebo JE, Khan N, Zabramski JM, Spetzler RF, editors. 16 Anesthetic and Perioperative Management of Moyamoya Disease. In: Moyamoya Disease [Internet]. Stuttgart: Georg Thieme Verlag; 2014 [cited 2021 Jan 20]. Available from: http://www.

thieme-connect.de/products/ebooks/abstract/10.1055/b-0034-92311

[46] Mariappan R, Mehta J, Chui J, Manninen P, Venkatraghavan L. Cerebrovascular reactivity to carbon dioxide under anesthesia: A qualitative systematic review [Internet]. Vol. 27, Journal of Neurosurgical Anesthesiology. Lippincott Williams and Wilkins; 2015 [cited 2021 Feb 6]. p. 123-35. Available from: https://journals.lww.com/00008506-201504000-00002

[47] Sumikawa K, Nagai H. Moyamoya disease and anesthesia [Internet]. Vol. 58, Anesthesiology. American Society of Anesthesiologists; 1983 [cited 2021 Jan 30]. p. 204-5. Available from: http://pubs.asahq.org/anesthesiology/article-pdf/58/2/204/306715/0000542-198302000-00033.pdf

[48] Li C, Zhang N, Yu S, Xu Y, Yao Y, Zeng M, et al. Individualized Perioperative Blood Pressure Management for Adult Moyamoya Disease: Experience from 186 Consecutive Procedures. J Stroke Cerebrovasc Dis. 2021 Jan 1;30(1).

[49] Kim SH, Choi JU, Yang KH, Kim TG, Kim DS. Risk factors for postoperative ischemic complications in patients with moyamoya disease. J Neurosurg [Internet]. 2005 Nov 1 [cited 2021 Jan 20];103 PEDIAT(SUPPL. 5):433-8. Available from: https://thejns.org/pediatrics/view/journals/j-neurosurg-pediatr/103/5/article-p433.xml

[50] Katsuki M, Fujimura M, Tashiro R, Tomata Y, Nishizawa T, Tominaga T. Pre-operative higher hematocrit and lower total protein levels are independent risk factors for cerebral hyperperfusion syndrome after superficial temporal artery–middle cerebral artery anastomosis with pial synangiosis in adult moyamoya disease patients—. Neurosurg Rev [Internet]. 2020 Sep 24 [cited 2021 Feb 6];1-10. Available from: https://link.springer.com/article/10.1007/s10143-020-01395-z

[51] Parray T, Martin TW, Siddiqui S. Moyamoya disease: A review of the disease and anesthetic management. Journal of Neurosurgical Anesthesiology. 2011.

[52] Ortiz-Cardona J, Bendo AA. Perioperative Pain Management in the Neurosurgical Patient. Vol. 25, Anesthesiology Clinics. 2007. p. 655-674.

[53] Vadivelu N, Kai AM, Tran D, Kodumudi G, Legler A, Ayrian E. Options for perioperative pain management in neurosurgery [Internet]. Vol. 9, Journal of Pain Research. Dove Medical Press Ltd.; 2016 [cited 2021 Jan 23]. p. 37-47. Available from: https://www.dovepress.com/options-for-perioperative-pain-management-in-neurosurgery-peer-reviewed-article-JPR

[54] Papangelou A, Radzik BR, Smith T, Gottschalk A. A review of scalp blockade for cranial surgery. Vol. 25, Journal of Clinical Anesthesia. Elsevier; 2013. p. 150-159.

[55] Geze S, Yilmaz AA, Tuzuner F. The effect of scalp block and local infiltration on the haemodynamic and stress response to skull-pin placement for craniotomy. Eur J Anaesthesiol [Internet]. 2009 Apr [cited 2021 Jan 30];26(4):298-303. Available from: http://journals.lww.com/00003643-200904000-00006

[56] Akhigbe T, Zolnourian A. Use of regional scalp block for pain management after craniotomy: Review of literature and critical appraisal of evidence. Vol. 45, Journal of Clinical Neuroscience. Churchill Livingstone; 2017. p. 44-47.

[57] Carella M, Tran G, Bonhomme VL, Franssen C. Influence of Levobupivacaine Regional Scalp Block on Hemodynamic Stability, Intra- and Postoperative

Opioid Consumption in Supratentorial Craniotomies: A Randomized Controlled Trial. Anesth Analg [Internet]. 2021 Feb [cited 2021 Jan 30];132(2):500-11. Available from: https://journals.lww.com/anesthesia-analgesia/Fulltext/2021/02000/Influence_of_Levobupivacaine_Regional_Scalp_Block.26.aspx

[58] Iwama T, Hashimoto N, Yonekawa Y. The relevance of hemodynamic factors to perioperative ischemic complications in childhood moyamoya disease. Neurosurgery [Internet]. 1996 Jun 1 [cited 2021 Jan 19];38(6):1120-6. Available from: https://academic.oup.com/neurosurgery/article/38/6/1120/2863840

[59] Sakamoto T, Kawaguchi M, Kurehara K, Kitaguchi K, Furuya H, Karasawa J. Risk Factors for Neurologic Deterioration After Revascularization Surgery in Patients with Moyamoya Disease. Anesth Analg. 1997 Nov;85(5):1060-1065.

[60] Zhao M, Deng X, Zhang D, Wang S, Zhang Y, Wang R, et al. Risk factors for and outcomes of postoperative complications in adult patients with moyamoya disease. J Neurosurg [Internet]. 2019 Feb 1 [cited 2021 Feb 6];130(2):531-42. Available from: https://thejns.org/doi/abs/10.3171/2017.10.JNS171749

[61] Powers WJ, Clarke WR, Grubb RL, Videen TO, Adams HP, Derdeyn CP. Extracranial-intracranial bypass surgery for stroke prevention in hemodynamic cerebral ischemia: The carotid occlusion surgery study randomized trial. JAMA - J Am Med Assoc. 2011;306(18):1983-92.

[62] Uno M, Nakajima N, Nishi K, Shinno K. Hyperperfusion Syndrome after Extracranial-Intracranial Bypass in a Patient with Moyamoya Disease: —Case Report—. Neurol Med Chir (Tokyo). 1998;38(7):420-424.

[63] Teo K, Choy DKS, Lwin S, Ning C, Yeo TT, Shen L, et al. Cerebral hyperperfusion syndrome after superficial temporal artery-middle cerebral artery bypass for severe intracranial steno-occlusive disease: A case control study. Neurosurgery. 2013;72(6):936-942.

[64] Fujimura M, Shimizu H, Inoue T, Mugikura S, Saito A, Tominaga T. Significance of focal cerebral hyperperfusion as a cause of transient neurologic deterioration after extracranial-intracranial bypass for moyamoya disease: Comparative study with non-moyamoya patients using n-isopropyl-p-[123I]iodoamphetamine single-phot. Neurosurgery. 2011;68(4):957-965.

[65] Yu J, Zhang J, Li J, Zhang J, Chen J. Cerebral Hyperperfusion Syndrome After Revascularization Surgery in Patients with Moyamoya Disease: Systematic Review and Meta-Analysis. Vol. 135, World Neurosurgery. Elsevier Inc.; 2020. p. 357-366.e4.

[66] Zhao WG, Luo Q, Jia JB, Yu JL. Cerebral hyperperfusion syndrome after revascularization surgery in patients with moyamoya disease. Vol. 27, British Journal of Neurosurgery. 2013. p. 321-325.

[67] Maragkos GA, Ascanio LC, Chida K, Boone MD, Ogilvy CS, Thomas AJ, et al. Moyamoya disease in pregnancy: a systematic review. Vol. 160, Acta Neurochirurgica. 2018. p. 1711-1719.

[68] Okutani R, Fukuhara A, Hino H, Shimada M, Kobayashi M. Anesthetic considerations during cesarean section procedures for two women with moyamoya disease - General vs subarachnoid anesthesia. Anesth Resusc. 2009;45(4):93-95.

[69] Abouleish E, Wiggins M, Ali V. Combined spinal and epidural anesthesia for cesarean section in a parturient with moyamoya

disease. Acta Anaesthesiol Scand. 1998;42(9):1120-1123.

[70] &NA; Anesthetic Management for Cesarean Section in Moyamoya Disease: A Report of Five Consecutive Cases and a Mini-Review. Obstet Anesth Dig. 2006;26(4):206-207.

[71] Inayama Y, Kondoh E, Chigusa Y, Io S, Funaki T, Matsumura N, et al. Moyamoya Disease in Pregnancy: A 20-Year Single-Center Experience and Literature Review. Vol. 122, World Neurosurgery. 2019. p. 684-691.e2.

[72] Gimovsky AC, Macri CJ, Bathgate SL, Ross DE. Moyamoya Disease in Pregnancy: Management after Intracranial Bypass Grafting. Case Rep Obstet Gynecol. 2012;2012:1-3.

[73] Irwin MG, Chung CKE, Ip KY, Wiles MD. Influence of propofol-based total intravenous anaesthesia on peri-operative outcome measures: a narrative review. Anaesthesia [Internet]. 2020 Jan 5 [cited 2021 Jan 20];75(S1):e90-100. Available from: https://onlinelibrary.wiley.com/doi/abs/10.1111/anae.14905

[74] Nakanishi T, Ukeda M, Toriumi T. Laparoscopic cholecystectomy in an adult moyamoya disease case. Vol. 35, Journal of Clinical Anesthesia. 2016. p. 240-241.

[75] Lim Y, Goel S, Brimacombe JR. The ProSeal™ laryngeal mask airway is an effective alternative to laryngoscope-guided tracheal intubation for gynaecological laparoscopy. Anaesth Intensive Care. 2007;35(1):52-56.

[76] Lee GY, Kim CH, Chung RK, Han JI. Intracranial hemorrhage during laparoscopic cholecystectomy due to unrecognized moyamoya disease. Vol. 27, Journal of Clinical Anesthesia. 2015. p. 81.

[77] Ishikawa S, Yamada T, Sakaguchi R, Hatorl E, Morisaki H. Anesthetic management of a patient with moyamoya disease undergoing mitral valve repair. Japanese J Anesthesiol. 2014;63(3):342-345.

[78] Okamoto K, Arai S, Hirabayashi N, Morita M, Kudo M, Yozu R, et al. Cerebral protection during mitral valve repair in a patient with moyamoya syndrome. Ann Thorac Surg. 2015;99(6):2208-2210.

[79] Saito K, Toyama H, Ejima Y, Yamauchi M. Anesthetic management in an adult moyamoya disease patient undergoing mitral valve plasty for severe mitral regurgitation. JA Clin Reports. 2016;2(1).

[80] Dulic G, Dulic I, Pozgain Z, Rimac M, Drinkovic M. Urgent off-pump coronary bypass grafting in moyamoya disease: A case report. Heart Surg Forum [Internet]. 2020 Mar 11 [cited 2021 Feb 6];23(2):E123-4. Available from: http://journal.hsforum.com

[81] Coşkun E, Altinay L, Tutun U, Tekin A. Off-pump coronary artery bypass grafting in moyamoya disease: A case report. Brazilian J Cardiovasc Surg. 2018;33(3):309-311.

Section 6

Treatment Options for Moyamoya Patients

Chapter 6

Medical Management in Moyamoya Disease

Nattaphol Uransilp, Sirinat Puengcharoen and Sombat Muengtaweepongsa

Abstract

Medical treatment seems to be not entirely helpful in the treatment of Moyamoya disease. No evidence supports the benefits of any drug treatment in Moyamoya disease. The ischemic or hemorrhagic event in Moyamoya disease is not preventable with any medical treatment. However, most of the physicians still prescribe the antithrombotic drug for Moyamoya patients with an ischemic event. Moreover, the standard guidelines recommend administering antithrombotic medications to treat Moyamoya with the ischemic event, even the risk of hemorrhagic complication. Antihypertensive drugs are routinely prescribed in Moyamoya patients with or without elevated blood pressure. A literature review about medical treatment in Moyamoya disease should help determine its use in this pathologic condition.

Keywords: Moyamoya disease, antithrombotic drugs, antiplatelet therapy, antihypertensive drugs, lipid-lowering drugs

1. Introduction

Moyamoya disease is a chronic steno-occlusive cerebrovascular disease characterized by progressive occlusion of bilateral distal ICA with a fine basal collateral network development. Long-term hemodynamic stress through the basal collateral network leads to cerebral ischemia and intracranial hemorrhage in children and adults, respectively. The study from Japan in 2007 reported the annual risk of any stroke as 3.2% in 34 non-surgically treated Moyamoya patients (mean follow up over 44 months) [1, 2].

Progressive stenosis of distal intracranial internal carotid arteries with a smoke-like appearance from collateral vessels in angiography is characteristic of Moyamoya disease [3]. The stenosis usually remains progressive until occlusion and flow diminish. Hemodynamic collapse is a primary mechanism for an ischemic event in Moyamoya disease. The preferred treatment for cerebral ischemia focuses on the correction of hemodynamic failure. This rationale makes surgical treatment essential, and medical management is not a principle for Moyamoya patients [4].

The name of moyamoya means puff of smoke, which refers to the collateral circulation's angiographic appearance. These collaterals are bundles of small, fragile arterioles that vulnerable to break out. The rupture of weak collateral vessels in Moyamoya disease is a primary mechanism for a hemorrhagic event. Revascularization surgery can reduce overload in collateral vessels, which prevents the vessels from getting ruptured [5]. In contrast, primary intracerebral hemorrhage is related to chronic hypertension [6]. The role of blood pressure control with antihypertensive drugs is not entirely clear for intracranial hemorrhage prevention in Moyamoya patients.

2. Methods

NU, SP, and SM independently search the Pubmed, MEDLINE, and Google Scholar for medical management in Moyamoya disease using the term "antithrombotic" or "antiplatelet" or "anticoagulant" or "thrombolytic" or "antihypertensive" or "lipid-lowering" or "aspirin" or "clopidogrel" or "cilostazol" or "warfarin" or "recombinant tissue plasminogen activator" and "Moyamoya."

2.1 The role of antithrombotic therapy in Moyamoya disease

Antithrombotic therapy consists of antiplatelet, anticoagulant, and thrombolytic agents. The rationale of antithrombotic is to prevent thrombogenesis [7]. It is not very confident that the ischemic event in Moyamoya disease is associated with thrombogenesis. The disease's pathogenesis lacks cerebral blood flow due to progressive stenosis of corresponding arteries rather than thrombo-embolism causes brain ischemia in Moyamoya patients. The role of antithrombotic therapy for ischemic prevention in Moyamoya disease is also not absolute.

However, hemodynamic failure may not be the only mechanism responsible for cerebral ischemia in Moyamoya disease. Larson et al. demonstrated that Moyamoya patients are predisposed to a pro-thrombotic state [8]. Shulman et al. reported evidence of artery-to-artery emboli in two separate Moyamoya cases. In the first patient, the emboli were visualized distally from the stenotic artery during bypass surgery. In the second case, the authors detected the emboli as a high-intensity transient signal (HITS) by transcranial Doppler (TCD) [9]. Jeon et al. reported the correlation between the emboli detected as HITS by TCD and the recent cerebral infarct [10]. The results of these two studies imply that hemodynamic compromise might not be the only mechanism for cerebral ischemia in Moyamoya patients. The evidence of artery-to-artery emboli opens up the role of antithrombotic therapy in Moyamoya disease. However, no clinical trial supports the use of antithrombotic drugs in Moyamoya disease.

Although there is no evidence to support clinical benefit, physicians still prescribe an antiplatelet agent as cerebral ischemic prevention in Moyamoya patients with symptomatic ischemic events or transient ischemic attacks (TIAs) [11, 12]. The single antiplatelet regimen with Aspirin is the most popular among the physicians. Most physicians prefer no antithrombotic treatment in asymptomatic Moyamoya patients [11]. Surgeons usually prescribe an antiplatelet agent after revascularization surgery [5, 11, 13–15]. After the surgery, antiplatelet treatment benefits include improving circulation to preserve cerebral perfusion, preventing small thrombus, and maintaining blood flow through surgical bypass [11, 14–16]. Aspirin remains the most popular antiplatelet agent prescribed by surgeons after surgery [15, 17]. Onozuka et al. reported that nearly 2,000 patients from Japan with non-hemorrhagic Moyamoya disease who received antiplatelet therapy before admission had better functional status than those who did not [18].

Other antiplatelet agents, such as Clopidogrel and Cilostazol, are also useful for ischemic prevention in Moyamoya disease [11]. Japanese and Korean physicians have the most experienced using Cilostazol in Moyamoya patients [19, 20]. Seo et al.'s upcoming report showed that nearly 10,000 patients from Korea who were prescribed antiplatelet benefited from reducing mortality, especially patients who received Cilostazol [21]. In contrast, Yamada et al. showed no benefit of antiplatelet treatment to prevent recurrent cerebral infarction in 344 Moyamoya patients with TIA or previous ischemic events in Japan [14].

The dual antiplatelet regimen has no role in Moyamoya disease, even in single regimen failure, due to the high risk for bleeding complications. The Japanese guidelines for Moyamoya disease management recommend using antiplatelet therapy as cerebral ischemic prevention, but with grade C level (can be considered, but adequate scientific rationale lacking) [22]. The long-term use of antiplatelet therapy for secondary ischemic prevention remains controversial because of the high risk for intracranial hemorrhage [12, 22].

The anticoagulants consist of the vitamin-K antagonist, heparin, low-molecular-weight heparin (LMWH), and non-vitamin-K antagonist. Due to the high risk of bleeding in Moyamoya disease, anticoagulants have no role in ischemic prevention, even in surgical or antiplatelet failure. Intravenous thrombolytic treatment with the recombinant tissue plasminogen activator (rtPA) is a standard treatment in acute ischemic stroke [23]. The Japanese guidelines for Moyamoya disease management recommend not giving the rtPA during acute ischemic stroke presentation due to the high risk of bleeding [22].

In summary, the single antiplatelet regimen with Aspirin, Clopidogrel, or Cilostazol may be useful for secondary ischemic prevention in Moyamoya patients with cerebral infarct or transient ischemic attack (TIA). The anticoagulants with the vitamin-K antagonist, heparin, low-molecular-weight heparin (LMWH), or non-vitamin-K antagonist have no role in Moyamoya patients. Intravenous rtPA has no role in Moyamoya patients with acute ischemic stroke. **Table 1** shows a summary of antithrombotic therapy in Moyamoya disease.

2.2 The role of antihypertensive treatment in Moyamoya disease

The Japanese guidelines for Moyamoya disease management recommend giving antihypertensive drugs to control blood pressure during the acute phase of intracranial hemorrhage for preventing hematoma expansion. However, the target blood pressure during the acute phase of intracranial hemorrhage is unclear. During the acute phase of intracranial hemorrhage in Moyamoya patients, the guidelines postulate that systolic and diastolic blood pressure should be under control below 180 and 105 mmHg, respectively, without any clinical evidence.

Comparing clinical outcomes between Moyamoya patients with and without hypertension in China shows that severe untreated hypertension is an independent risk factor for unfavorable outcomes [24]. Antihypertensive drugs could prevent patients with hypertension from unfavorable outcomes. Long term antihypertensive treatment is only for Moyamoya patients with hypertension. The target blood

Antithrombotic treatment	The role of treatment in Moyamoya disease
Antiplatelet	Secondary prevention for cerebral ischemia Agents: Aspirin (50–325 mg) Clopidogrel (75 mg) Cilostazol (200 mg)
Anticoagulant	No role
Thrombolysis	No role

Table 1.
The role of antithrombotic treatment in Moyamoya disease.

Antihypertensive treatment	The role of treatment in Moyamoya disease
• Nicardipine 5–15 mg/hour • Labetalol 10 mg IV over 1–2 minutes followed by infusion of 2–8 mg/min	The acute phase of intracranial hemorrhage
• Angiotensin-converting enzyme inhibitors • Angiotensin receptor blockers • Calcium channel blockers (highly lipophilic) • Diuretics	Presenting concurrent hypertension: secondary prevention for cerebral ischemia or hemorrhage

Table 2.
The role of antihypertensive treatment in Moyamoya disease.

Lipid-lowering therapy	The role of treatment in Moyamoya disease
• Statins	Presenting concurrent dyslipidemia (LDL > 100)

Table 3.
The role of lipid-lowering therapy in Moyamoya disease.

pressure for Moyamoya patients with chronic hypertension should refer to which recommended in standard guidelines for hypertension. The fisrt-line antihypertensive drugs recommended by the guidelines include Angiotensin-converting enzyme inhibitors, Angiotensin receptor blockers, Calcium channel blockers and Diuretics [25]. Routine use of antihypertensive drugs in Moyamoya patients without hypertension for primary hemorrhagic or ischemic prevention is not recommended [22]. **Table 2** shows the role of antihypertensive treatment in Moyamoya disease.

2.3 The role of lipid-lowering therapy in Moyamoya disease

The benefit of lipid-lowering treatment in Moyamoya disease is unclear. There is no direct clinical trial regarding lipid-lowering therapy in Moyamoya disease. Among those lipid-lowering drugs, statins are the only sub-group that give benefit for primary and secondary ischemic stroke prevention in patients with presumed atherosclerotic disease [26, 27]. The indirect evidence from Church et al.'s study demonstrated that statins, the essential lipid-lowering drugs for atherosclerosis treatment, may reduce unilateral Moyamoya disease progression [28]. The Japanese guidelines for Moyamoya disease management do not recommend routine prescribing lipid-lowering treatment, except for presenting concurrent dyslipidemia [22]. It is reasonable to lower the low-density lipopretien (LDL) below 100 mg/dL as recommended in stroke patients with presumed atherosclerotic disease (**Table 3**).

3. Summary

Antiplatelet treatment with a single agent regimen is useful for Moyamoya patients with cerebral ischemia. There is no role of neither anticoagulant nor thrombolytic therapy in Moyamoya disease. Moyamoya patients with hypertension should get antihypertensive treatment. Experts do not recommend routinely prescribing antihypertensive drugs in Moyamoya disease without hypertension. Moyamoya patients with dyslipidemia may gain benefit from lipid-lowering therapy.

Acknowledgements

This study is supported by the Center of Excellence in Stroke from Thammasat University.

Author details

Nattaphol Uransilp, Sirinat Puengcharoen and Sombat Muengtaweepongsa*
Center of Excellence in Stroke, Faculty of Medicine, Thammasat University, Pathum Thani, 12120, Thailand

*Address all correspondence to: sombatm@hotmail.com

References

[1] Kim JS. Moyamoya Disease: Epidemiology, Clinical Features, and Diagnosis. J Stroke. 2016;18(1):2-11.

[2] Kim T, Oh CW, Bang JS, Kim JE, Cho WS. Moyamoya Disease: Treatment and Outcomes. J Stroke. 2016;18(1):21-30.

[3] Gupta A, Tyagi A, Romo M, Amoroso KC, Sonia F. Moyamoya Disease: A Review of Current Literature. Cureus. 2020.

[4] Kossorotoff M, Tournier-Lasserve E, Herve D, Guey S. Moyamoya disease and syndromes: from genetics to clinical management. The Application of Clinical Genetics. 2015:49.

[5] Houkin K, Kamiyama H, Abe H, Takahashi A, Kuroda S. Surgical Therapy for Adult Moyamoya Disease. Stroke. 1996;27(8):1342-6.

[6] Thabet AM, Kottapally M, Hemphill Iii JC. Chapter 11 - Management of intracerebral hemorrhage. In: Eelco FMW, Andreas HK, editors. Handbook of Clinical Neurology. Volume 140: Elsevier; 2017. p. 177-94.

[7] Blann AD, Landray MJ, Lip GYH. An overview of antithrombotic therapy. BMJ. 2002;325(7367):762-5.

[8] Larson A, Rinaldo L, Lanzino G, Klaas JP. High prevalence of pro-thrombotic conditions in adult patients with moyamoya disease and moyamoya syndrome: a single center study. Acta Neurochir (Wien). 2020;162(8):1853-9.

[9] Shulman JG, Snider S, Vaitkevicius H, Babikian VL, Patel NJ. Direct Visualization of Arterial Emboli in Moyamoya Syndrome. Front Neurol. 2017;8:425.

[10] Jeon C, Yeon JY, Jo KI, Hong SC, Kim JS. Clinical Role of Microembolic Signals in Adult Moyamoya Disease With Ischemic Stroke. Stroke. 2019;50(5):1130-5.

[11] Oki K, Katsumata M, Izawa Y, Takahashi S, Suzuki N, Houkin K, et al. Trends of Antiplatelet Therapy for the Management of Moyamoya Disease in Japan: Results of a Nationwide Survey. J Stroke Cerebrovasc Dis. 2018;27(12):3605-12.

[12] Kraemer M, Berlit P, Diesner F, Khan N. What is the expert's option on antiplatelet therapy in moyamoya disease? Results of a worldwide Survey. European Journal of Neurology. 2012;19(1):163-7.

[13] Agarwalla PK, Stapleton CJ, Phillips MT, Walcott BP, Venteicher AS, Ogilvy CS. Surgical outcomes following encephaloduroarteriosynangiosis in North American adults with moyamoya. J Neurosurg. 2014;121(6):1394-400.

[14] Yamada S, Oki K, Itoh Y, Kuroda S, Houkin K, Tominaga T, et al. Effects of Surgery and Antiplatelet Therapy in Ten-Year Follow-Up from the Registry Study of Research Committee on Moyamoya Disease in Japan. J Stroke Cerebrovasc Dis. 2016;25(2):340-9.

[15] Zhao Y, Zhang Q, Zhang D, Zhao Y. Effect of Aspirin in Postoperative Management of Adult Ischemic Moyamoya Disease. World Neurosurgery. 2017;105:728-31.

[16] Zakeri AS, Nimjee SM. Use of Antiplatelet Agents in the Neurosurgical Patient. Neurosurg Clin N Am. 2018;29(4):517-27.

[17] Schubert GA, Biermann P, Weiss C, Seiz M, Vajkoczy P, Schmiedek P, et al. Risk Profile In Extracranial/Intracranial Bypass Surgery—The Role of Antiplatelet Agents, Disease Pathology, and Surgical Technique In 168 Direct

Revascularization Procedures. World Neurosurgery. 2014;82(5):672-7.

[18] Onozuka D, Hagihara A, Nishimura K, Kada A, Nakagawara J, Ogasawara K, et al. Prehospital antiplatelet use and functional status on admission of patients with non-haemorrhagic moyamoya disease: a nationwide retrospective cohort study (J-ASPECT study). BMJ Open. 2016;6(3):e009942.

[19] Chiba T, Setta K, Shimada Y, Yoshida J, Fujimoto K, Tsutsui S, et al. Comparison of Effects between Clopidogrel and Cilostazol on Cerebral Perfusion in Nonsurgical Adult Patients with Symptomatically Ischemic Moyamoya Disease: Subanalysis of a Prospective Cohort. J Stroke Cerebrovasc Dis. 2018;27(11):3373-9.

[20] Ando S, Tsutsui S, Miyoshi K, Sato S, Yanagihara W, Setta K, et al. Cilostazol may improve cognition better than clopidogrel in non-surgical adult patients with ischemic moyamoya disease: subanalysis of a prospective cohort. Neurological Research. 2019;41(5):480-7.

[21] Seo W-K, Kim J-Y, Eun-Hyeok C, Kim Y-S, Chung J-W, Saver JL, et al. Association of Antiplatelet Therapy, Including Cilostazol, with Improved Survival in Patients with Moyamoya Disease in a Nationwide Study. The Lancet Neurology. 2019.

[22] Guidelines for Diagnosis and Treatment of Moyamoya Disease (Spontaneous Occlusion of the Circle of Willis). Neurologia medico-chirurgica. 2012;52(5):245-66.

[23] Powers William J, Rabinstein Alejandro A, Ackerson T, Adeoye Opeolu M, Bambakidis Nicholas C, Becker K, et al. Guidelines for the Early Management of Patients With Acute Ischemic Stroke: 2019 Update to the 2018 Guidelines for the Early Management of Acute Ischemic Stroke: A Guideline for Healthcare Professionals From the American Heart Association/American Stroke Association. Stroke. 2019;50(12):e344-e418.

[24] Ma Y, Zhao M, Deng X, Zhang D, Wang S, Zeng Z, et al. Comparison of clinical outcomes and characteristics between patients with and without hypertension in moyamoya disease. J Clin Neurosci. 2020;75:163-7.

[25] James PA, Oparil S, Carter BL, Cushman WC, Dennison-Himmelfarb C, Handler J, et al. 2014 evidence-based guideline for the management of high blood pressure in adults: report from the panel members appointed to the Eighth Joint National Committee (JNC 8). JAMA. 2014;311(5):507-20.

[26] Meschia JF, Bushnell C, Boden-Albala B, Braun LT, Bravata DM, Chaturvedi S, et al. Guidelines for the primary prevention of stroke: a statement for healthcare professionals from the American Heart Association/American Stroke Association. Stroke. 2014;45(12):3754-832.

[27] Kernan WN, Ovbiagele B, Black HR, Bravata DM, Chimowitz MI, Ezekowitz MD, et al. Guidelines for the Prevention of Stroke in Patients With Stroke and Transient Ischemic Attack. Stroke. 2014;45(7):2160-236.

[28] Church EW, Bell-Stephens TE, Bigder MG, Gummidipundi S, Han SS, Steinberg GK. Clinical Course of Unilateral Moyamoya Disease. Neurosurgery. 2020;87(6):1262-8.

Chapter 7

Surgical Treatment of Moyamoya Disease

Vicente Vanaclocha, Nieves Saiz-Sapena and Leyre Vanaclocha

Abstract

Moyamoya disease is a rare cerebrovascular disease most prevalent in East Asian Countries. Thanks to the new diagnostic capabilities, the number of cases discovered has been rising steadily in the latest years, including many asymptomatic patients. But asymptomatic from the clinical point of view does not necessarily mean that there are no subjacent problems and that there will be no disease progression. Indeed, many patients harbour cognitive decline long before they start with clinical or even radiological manifestations. The only effective treatment is surgical revascularization, with all its possibilities: direct, indirect, and combined. While direct techniques are more useful in adult moyamoya patients, children seem to benefit most from indirect techniques. Additionally, indirect or combined procedures can be used as salvage procedures in case of unsatisfactory outcomes. Thus, many surgeons posit that surgical treatment should be considered in moyamoya patients, even if asymptomatic, particularly in the paediatric age group.

Keywords: moyamoya disease, surgical revascularization, bypass surgery, asymptomatic moyamoya disease, cerebral revascularization, treatments modalities

1. Introduction

Takeuchi and Shimizu first described Moyamoya disease (MMD) in 1957 [1]. It is an idiopathic cerebral vasculopathy characterised by progressive stenosis of the terminal internal carotid artery and its branches, usually on both sides, and the development of a compensatory network of abnormal collateral vessels [2]. Unilateral involvement does not rule out this disease [3]. It affects mainly the middle (MCA) and anterior cerebral (ACA) arteries, less commonly the posterior cerebral or the middle meningeal arteries, and in a few cases the arteries that supply other organs [4], like the lungs or kidneys [5]. Some MMD patients suffer from pulmonary artery hypertension, which usually starts in adolescence or young adulthood and progresses slowly [5].

The collateral vessels that develop as the disease progresses [6] have a thin and weak non-elastic wall with aneurysm formation prone to haemorrhages [7–9]. These aneurysms' prevalence varies in the different series between 1.9 [10], 2.8% [11], 3.9 [12], 8.3 [6] and 14% [13]. They are usually located in deep areas [11], small in size and with very fragile walls, making their treatment, endovascular or surgical, extremely challenging [11, 12, 14]. They can also be found at the circle of Willis [9, 11, 15, 16], where they usually have a fusiform shape [11, 17] and can lead to a subarachnoid haemorrhage [11]. The prognosis in the case of this type of haemorrhage is poor [11].

Their recommended treatment is brain revascularization (BR) [12, 18, 19] as many regress spontaneously after their haemodynamic stress is reduced [11, 20–24].

MMD can be associated with other diseases like Down syndrome (trisomy 21) [25], sickle cell disease [26], neurofibromatosis type 1 [27], thalassemia [28], Graves' disease [29] and after head- and neck-radiotherapy [30]. In this case, it is known as moyamoya syndrome [3].

MMD patients have impaired cerebral haemodynamics with a low cerebral blood flow (CBF) or a poor brain vasodilatory capacity, making them prone to cerebrovascular events [31], particularly at the frontal lobe [32]. The CBF and the cerebral vascular reserve (CVR) capacity are used to evaluate the need for surgical treatment [33–36].

Although it is a rare disease, it is the leading cause of ischemic stroke in the paediatric population in Korea and Japan [37–39].

Digital subtraction angiography (DSA) is the gold standard for diagnosis, but Magnetic Resonance Angiography (MRA) is also helpful [40, 41]. More specific methods but not currently used because of the costs and equipment involved are xenon-enhanced CT, DSC, MRI, H_2[^{15}O]-PET and [42] I aromatic amines SPECT [43–48]. These diagnostic techniques are used for preoperative evaluation to decide the best surgical approach. Their drawbacks are that they require contrast agents' intravenous injection and entail radiation exposure that can be harmful to patients, particularly in the paediatric age group. Preoperative transcranial colour-duplex sonography is a non-invasive method used to evaluate the degree of vascular impairment in MMD and monitor the results after surgical BR [49–51].

The patients' mean age at diagnosis peaks at ten and 30–50 years [9, 12, 52] with a ratio of women-to-men 1.00:1.03 [12].

MMD two basic clinical manifestation types are ischemic (30.4%) and haemorrhagic (70.9%) stroke [12]. The ischemic type is more common in children and the haemorrhagic in adults [13, 53]. Other clinical symptoms are headache [54], epilepsy [55], chorea movements [56] and cognitive decline [53, 57]. In comparison, haemorrhages are more frequent in the adult MMD population [58] and ischemic events in the paediatric age group [59–62]. Patients starting with ischemic symptoms like transitory ischemic attack (TIA) are more prone to develop an ischemic than a haemorrhagic stroke [63, 64]. In the paediatric population, multiple ischemic strokes, significantly if both hemispheres are affected, can lead to severe cognitive impairment and developmental delay [65–67]. Brain infarcts present in the ACA and MCA territories and less commonly in the posterior cerebral artery (PCA) covered area and vertebrobasilar system [68]. Posterior circulation involvement leads to more severe symptomatology and worse outcomes [69]. Haemorrhagic strokes are often followed by rebleeding and infarction in short to medium follow-up [70].

Unless surgical BR is undertaken, the stroke rate is 18% for the first year and 3.2–5% for the following years [71–73]. Once patients suffer an ischemic or haemorrhagic stroke, the risk of a new cerebrovascular insult in the following five years is 65% [74, 75].

In MMD, the PCA provides the collateral flow to the anterior circulation [32, 76–79] with choroidal anastomosis and hypertrophic collateral vessel formation [76, 80]. This increased blood flow through the PCA creates haemodynamic stress on the vertebrobasilar system and facilitates aneurysm formation [76, 81]. The choroidal collateral vessels are potential sources of haemorrhages and rebleeding [82]. A common complication is a brain haemorrhage [80, 83, 84], usually intraventricular [80, 85], particularly in the rear brain areas [80]. Moreover, MMD patients with haemorrhages in the posterior part of the brain have a higher risk of rebleeding than those with haemorrhages located in the anterior part [85]. PCA stenosis is typical of juvenile-onset MMD [86].

Microbleeds' are more common in MMD than in the general population [87] and usually in the periventricular areas, followed by the basal ganglia and thalamus [87–89]. The asymptomatic microbleeds are related to hypertrophy, dilatation and aneurysm formation of the posterior communicating and anterior choroidal arteries [90–92]. Those areas are where the MMD related haemorrhagic strokes typically happen, and these microbleeds are an excellent prognosticator of future haemorrhages [83, 93, 94].

Asymptomatic MMD patients have a 3.2% annual stroke risk [95], more often haemorrhagic than ischemic, showing an evolving situation that is usually is not silent nor stable [72, 96], particularly in those with a compromised CVR capacity [97]. Moreover, cognitive decline over time is the rule [98]. Thus, asymptomatic MMD patients should be monitored closely and submitted to surgical BR at the slightest sign of deterioration [99].

Although there might be a subgroup of children with a benign course [100], most have a relentless and progressive worsening [99], and unilateral disease often evolves to bilateral [99]. Predictors of unfavourable outcome are onset at a younger age, a long time before BR, brain infarcts, and PCA involvement [86]. Children under nine years of age with minor changes in the contralateral brain hemisphere are most likely to undergo disease progression [101, 102].

This disease, particularly if untreated, can induce severe disability and even death [3]. White matter involvement, particularly in adults, correlates with cognitive impairment [57].

2. Treatment modalities in moyamoya disease

Without a known aetiology, the only treatment is symptomatic. The medical treatment does not affect this disease's relentless progression [103, 104], and patients under drug treatment alone have a 5-year 65% stroke risk [72, 105–107] which climbs up to a dismal 82% in case of bilateral involvement [105]. In children, it has been reported that under conservative treatment, 37% will present clinical symptoms of neurological damage, and 3% will eventually die [108]. It can be helpful, though, to alleviate some symptoms like headache or epileptic seizures [109]. Endovascular treatment has been attempted in some cases with unsatisfactory results [110–112]. The surgical treatment with BR offloads the haemodynamic stress [113] and reduces the risk of subsequent ischemic and haemorrhagic cerebrovascular events [104, 114–122], providing symptom improvement to 87% of patients [104].

BR techniques can be classified into two main groups: direct and indirect. The first involves artery-to-artery bypasses between an external carotid artery branch and a brain arterial vessel, usually between the superficial temporal (STA) and MCA [42, 115, 123]. Other donor vessels are the occipital [69, 124], deep temporal, and middle meningeal [125] arteries. The STA can be connected to a branch of the middle cerebral [126] or anterior cerebral [127] arteries. Meanwhile, the occipital artery is sutured to the PCA [128] but can also be used to revascularize the MCA territory [129]. The size of the donor artery should be >0.8 mm to allow the surgical manoeuvres [130]. In children under four years of age, both the STA and the possible recipient brain arteries usually have an insufficient diameter to enable a bypass [131]. Its most significant advantage is that it provides immediate brain haemodynamic improvement. This fast improvement in the brain blood flow reduces the risk of ischemic and haemorrhagic strokes faster than the indirect techniques, which require 3–4 months to achieve the same result [132]. Its main risk is a hyperperfusion-reperfusion syndrome, which can induce haemorrhages with neurological deterioration and worsening [115, 133, 134]. This risk can be minimised with strict postoperative blood pressure control and mild hypotension in symptomatic cerebral hyperperfusion [135]. Direct BR is mainly used to increase the perfusion of the MCA territory [99]. Direct BR of the anterior or PCA branches is challenging as the donor's vessels are further away, a severe problem when those vascular territories are affected [99]. Under experienced hands, the patency rates are over 90% [136]. As the cortical arteries atrophy, it is increasingly difficult to find a suitable recipient vessel to perform a direct bypass [137]. The ideal is an M_3 branch, but micro-anastomoses with these vessels are technically very difficult [138].

In the indirect BR, no arterial anastomoses are performed. Instead, a pedicle graft vascularized by the external carotid artery is placed over the brain's surface and rely on the new collateral vessel formation between the donor tissue and the ischemic underlying brain [139]. For a successful result, three elements are needed—first, a well-vascularized donor tissue. Second, intimate contact between donor tissue and recipient brain vascularization. And third, a good selection of the hypoperfused recipient brain areas [140]. Indirect BR requires forming a fibrous scar at the donor tissue-brain interface with new collateral vessel formation between the donor and recipient vascular beds [141]. The possibilities of indirect BR techniques are broad [104]. Depending on the donor tissue used, the options are encephalo-myo-synangiosis (EMS) [142] when a muscle is used, encephalo-duro-synangiosis (EDS) [143] with dural graft, split-duro-encephalo-synangiosis (DES) [144, 145] with a split dura graft, encephalo-duro-myo-synangiosis (EDMS) [146] with dural and muscle graft, encephalo-duro-arterio-synangiosis (EDAS) [147–150] with dura and external carotid artery branch, encephalo-duro-arterio-myo-synagiosis (EDAMS) [151] with dura, an external carotid artery branch and muscle, encephalo-galeo-synangiosis (EGS) [152, 153] with galea, encephalo-pericranium-synangiosis (EPS) [140, 154, 155] with pericranium, omentum transplantation [156, 157] and multiple burr-hole (MBH) [158, 159]. This last surgical technique consists of performing numerous burr holes (10 to 24) through the frontal, parietal and occipital bones, opening the dura and arachnoid and introducing a pericranium flap inside each burr-hole [160]. It can be used isolated, as part of other BR techniques or as a rescue procedure when other surgical approaches have failed or proved insufficient [160–162]. Not only is it technically effortless and straightforward, but it can be performed under local anaesthesia, which is an advantage in patients in a seriously compromised status [161]. As the dura is also an essential source of collateral vessel formation, a small craniotomy (3–3.5 cm in diameter) placing the pericranium directly over the brain surface provides better results than MBH [140]. Contrarywise, extensive craniotomies are not recommended because they disrupt the already spontaneously formed collateral vascularization increasing the risk of postoperative brain ischemic events [140]. The EPS is particularly helpful to provide collateral circulation to the anterior and PCA territories, areas not easily covered by the STA [140]. Duropexy is crucial in all indirect BR techniques [140].

Direct BR is preferred whenever possible because the haemodynamically compromised hemisphere gets an immediate increase in blood flow, reducing sooner the ischemic and haemorrhagic stroke risk [113, 163]. In contrast, with the indirect techniques, the new collateral vascularization takes 3 to 4 months to develop [53, 164, 165], but long-term, the blood–brain supply is better than with the direct BR [141]. In this period in which the collateral vessel formation is taking place, may persist brain hypoperfusion symptoms, and at times the final result may require an additional surgical BR procedure [128, 166–168].

With the direct bypass, the brain perfusion improvement is limited to the area where it is undertaken and is not helpful to perfuse extensive ischemic areas [169].

Contrarywise indirect brain vascularization can cover vast vascular territories, mainly if different techniques are employed, like the EDAS combined with MBH [5, 159]. This combination can provide new blood supply to the whole brain, including the interhemispheric frontal areas and occipital lobe [68].

MMD related aneurysms were treated with embolization or surgical clipping [11], and many improved with BR alone [11, 12].

3. Historical development of surgical BR for MMD

Yaşargil performed the first superficial-temporal artery bypass procedure for an MMD patient in 1972 [170]. In Japan, the first case was completed in 1973 by Kikuchi and Karasawa [171]. In the following years, Karasawa and colleagues in Japan refined this surgical procedure and reported their results in 1978 [123].

The first indirect MMD BR was reported by Karasawa in 1977 and was called encephalo-myo-synangiosis (EMS) [142]. Several researchers confirmed that placement of the temporalis muscle directly over the brain induced collateral vessel formation [172–174]. In 1980 Matsushima et al. introduced a new indirect BR technique, the EDAS [175]. The STA with a strip of its surrounding galea was placed directly over the brain through a linear dural incision [176]. The galea was sutured to the dural edges, and the STA left over the brain without interrupting its flow, waiting for collateral vessel formation between the dura, the galea, the STA and the brain. It became widely accepted [149, 153, 177–180]. The EMS was the ground stone for other indirect BR techniques introduced in the following years that used different donor tissues, including other scalp arteries [177], split dura [145], neck [181] or distant [182–184] muscles and the omentum [156]. Others reported using the pericranium introduced though multiple burr-holes [185]. These techniques revascularized the MCA territory but not those of the anterior and posterior cerebral arteries. In 1992, Inoue et al. [186] introduced the frontal EDAMS to selectively revascularize the anterior cerebral bed to overcome this drawback. Kinugasa et al. [187] two years later reported the ribbon EDAMS, in which a strip of galea and pericranium were placed over the frontal lobes, including the interhemispheric areas. Tenjin et al. [177] published in 1997 the occipital artery's use to revascularize the PCA territory. Ever since a combination of direct and indirect BR techniques is recommended to achieve a good collateral flow in all three brain arterial territories (anterior, middle, and posterior cerebral arteries).

4. Indication of surgical techniques for cerebral revascularization in moyamoya disease

The hemisphere with the worse vascularization is operated first [12]. If both hemispheres are equally affected, the recommendation is to start with the dominant one and revascularize the other six months latter [178].

In unilateral involvement, if the patients' symptoms disappear with the unilateral BR and an asymptomatic contralateral hemisphere, no further brain vascularization is advised for the time being [12] as contralateral hemisphere surgical BR in patients with unilateral involvement is controversial [99]. In an ischemic or haemorrhagic stroke, surgical BR is delayed for at least six weeks [188], and ideally, three months [12] and the BR of the contralateral cerebral hemisphere postponed at least 4–6 weeks [148]. Nevertheless, delaying surgical treatment is not advisable in late Suzuki stages [2], as BR improves brain collateral vascularization but not the stroke rate [178]. So, once the diagnosis is made, it is better to avoid unnecessary delays, particularly in children [178].

Direct BR is particularly indicated in adult and adolescent MMD patients [189, 190] but not recommended before ten years of age [191]. An STA to MCA bypass is strongly advised as it corrects the MMD related hemodynamic insufficiency [71, 121]. For a successful result, both the donor and recipient arteries must be at least 0.8 mm in outer diameter [192].

Indirect techniques are much less demanding [193] but are not as valuable for adults as for children [99, 149, 150, 152, 159, 179, 194, 195]. Its main drawback is that BR takes time, on average 3–4 months [196], during which there is a continued risk of cerebrovascular events [140]. In the paediatric age group, these indirect surgical techniques are preferred because the vessels are often of insufficient size and maturity to safely allow a direct arterial bypass [197], significantly below ten years of age [198]. One of the main advantages of indirect BR is the possibility of improving the anterior and PAC territories' blood perfusion apart from the area covered by the MCA [146, 199]. This possibility of a wider area covered by the BR is crucial in children [99, 152, 158] as they often develop long-term symptoms secondary to hypoperfusion of the whole hemisphere [99]. The BR that use the temporalis muscle is not recommended in children [200] because it thickens with time, compressing the brain and inducing ischemia [201] and because it adheres to the brain and when it contracts can cause long-term neurological damage [202]. Additionally, it generates an unsightly cosmetic head [200].

A combination of direct and indirect BR procedures is often used to profit from the advantages of each of them [34, 114, 136, 150, 160, 203], because the reported results are better than isolated direct or indirect techniques [204–207]. The treatment strategy has to be tailored to the specific needs of each patient [136, 160, 208]. Combining more than one indirect BR techniques has similar mortality and morbidity as any of them isolated [136].

During the surgical procedure, it is essential to avoid hypotension, hyperthermia, hypocarbia, hypercarbia, and epileptic seizures as they all increase the brain metabolism and thus the chance of an ischemic event [148, 149, 188, 200, 209–211] and perioperative morbidity [212]. It is vital to control the pain and cry in the postoperative period to avoid hyperventilation as this will produce hypocarbia and an increased risk of ischemia [149, 213]. It is recommended to provide intravenous fluids at 1.5 times the regular maintenance rate for 48–72 hours [3, 149]. Platelet counts and prothrombin time must be monitored and controlled with transfusions if needed [148]. The blood haemoglobin must be kept above the 12–13 g/dL range [148].

Some improvements in the surgical technique have eased the surgical manoeuvres and improved the clinical results. Among them is placing 10-0 Proline sutures to the arachnoid membrane in both sides of the brain sulcus. When some retraction is applied, the recipient artery is brought to the surface, and the STA to MCA bypass is made more easily [192].

While it seems intuitive that arachnoid removal will improve the collateral vessel formation between the donor artery or tissue and the brain [153], it is no longer recommended in indirect BR because it is associated with a significantly higher complication risk with no improvement in the final clinical outcome [148]. Among these complications are the postoperative ischemic strokes secondary to the vasospasm induced by the arachnoid dissection [148]. Preserving the arachnoid membrane reduces the operating time at an average of 30 minutes [148].

The middle meningeal artery provides a vital source of collateral circulation, so during the surgical procedure, this artery and its main branches should be preserved as much as possible [191]. Preservation of this crucial source of collateral vessel formation requires gentle dura handling and careful planning of any dural incisions.

Some have recommended medical treatment for asymptomatic MMD because it is associated with a 5.3% rate of clinical progression [97] unless they have reduced cerebral vascular reserve [97, 103, 214] or smoke [97, 215]. Most of these asymptomatic patients will undergo disease progression [103, 216]. When that happens, surgical BR is advisable [95, 103, 215].

In case of failure to initial BR, a new procedure, direct, indirect or combined, should be attempted, as good outcomes are common [166, 217].

5. Results surgical techniques of cerebral revascularization in moyamoya disease

BR decreased both the haemorrhagic [115] and the ischemic stroke [164, 218], but it is more effective in the first than in the second [219–221]. On one-year follow-up, haemorrhagic stroke was 4.6% for those who underwent BR versus 18.6% for those managed conservatively [115, 116, 164, 219]. The mortality rate due to haemorrhagic stroke is four times higher in the conservative than in the BR group [116, 164, 220]. The medical treatment had even worse results in the paediatric than in the adult MMD age group [107, 222].

Younger age at BR surgery correlates with better results and long-term prognosis [62, 164, 205]. In children, indirect BR is associated with a 0.4%/year symptomatic haemorrhage and 0.2%/year infarction rates, with cumulative incidences of 1.8% at ten, 7.3% at 20 and 7.3% at 30 years [223, 224]. There are no statistically significative differences in clinical outcome between direct, indirect and combined BR procedures [99, 205]. The average good clinical outcome is 84.8–88% [143, 205] with a 6.4% 5-year risk of ischemic or haemorrhagic stroke [143]. Children seem to improve more than adults (93% versus 82.7%) [205].

Direct BR with extra-intracranial artery bypass significantly decreases the haemorrhagic stroke rate [115, 223], particularly in the patients with haemorrhages in the posterior half of the brain [85]. Compared to indirect procedures, it reduces the stroke risk [116, 205, 219, 221], particularly the haemorrhagic type in adults [225] and adolescents [196]. These differences are not so evident in children as adults due to the technical difficulty in performing a successful arterial bypass in the first group [140]. Both in adults and the paediatric population, direct BR is technically more challenging that indirect BR, demands a longer operating time, and there is always the risk of hyperperfusion syndrome [116]. There no statistically significative difference in the number of perioperative complications between direct and indirect BR techniques [219]. The direct bypass was accompanied by an annual stroke rate of 0–6% for children and 1.4% for adults, while the indirect techniques had a 1.6% stroke rate for the same period of time [196]. Direct BR is recommended whenever it is technically feasible [197, 221].

Indirect BR is easier to perform, but 40–50% of adult MMD patients do not develop an adequate collateral arterial circulation [53, 62, 141, 226]. These results have been improved with changes in the surgical technique and perioperative care [140], but a new surgical procedure with a combined approach will be needed if there is an unsatisfactory outcome [189, 207, 224]. Meanwhile, paediatric patients submitted to indirect BR have low middle and long term haemorrhagic stroke rates [227, 228].

Perioperative complications happen in 9.4–13.6% of BR procedures [116, 149, 194, 205, 219, 221, 226] with a 0–0.5% [188] mortality rate. Indirect BR has a significantly higher postoperative stroke rate than direct techniques [116, 205] but fewer haemorrhages and no hyperperfusion syndrome [140, 229, 230]. The incidence of postoperative surgical complications is higher in Asian than other racial groups (6.51/100,00 inhabitants/year versus 5.21/100,000/persons/year) [198, 231]. They also show a different response to BR [198]. Patients with MMD associated with other diseases have a higher perioperative complication rate than regular MMD patients [188].

Preoperative infarction is related to a greater risk of postoperative complications [232, 233].

Direct or combined BR is associated with better outcomes than indirect BR, particularly in the ischemic type MMD [140, 190, 205]. Meanwhile, for haemorrhagic strokes, there are no differences between direct, indirect or combined BR, and thus the indirect techniques are recommended because they are more accessible to perform [205].

The best collateral vessel formation results are obtained using a superficial temporal to MCA bypass combined with an EDAMS and lowest with EDAS [140]. Nevertheless, EDAS combined with multiple burr-holes can provide similar outcomes with a less technically demanding procedure and fewer postoperative negative events [159, 177].

Surgical BR in MMD can prevent future cerebrovascular insults and avoid cognitive decline [116, 117, 227]. It is indicated in asymptomatic patients at the slightest sign of disease progression or patient neurological or mental impairment [103, 234, 235], particularly in the paediatric age group [62, 103]. If performed early before irreversible damage, it can improve the neurological status and prevent the cognitive decline [103], stopping or at least slowing the progression of this nasty disease [136, 206, 234]. Ideally, in children, the surgical BR should be performed not later than three months after the first symptoms appear at a young age [190], the best before six years of age [106].

6. Conclusions

MMD is an uncommon cerebrovascular disorder with a higher frequency among people with Asian ancestry. Medical treatment is not helpful to stop the MMD progression and only can control minor symptoms but not ischemic nor haemorrhagic events. BR can improve brain vascularization, providing a collateral blood supply source that contains this nasty disease's progression. Direct BR is more effective in adults and adolescents than in the paediatric population. Children benefit most from indirect BR. Combined BR improves the results from direct and indirect BR and can also be used as a rescue procedure. Although controversial, many surgeons posit that asymptomatic MMD patients should be submitted to preventive BR before irreversible brain damage happens.

Abbreviations

ACA	anterior cerebral artery
BR	brain revascularization
CBF	cerebral blood flow
CVR	cerebral vascular reserve
DES	split-duro-encephalo-synangiosis
EDS	encephalo-duro-synangiosis
EDAMS	encephalo-duro-arterio-myo-synagiosis
EDAS	encephalo-duro-arterio-synangiosis
EDMS	encephalo-duro-myo-synangiosis

EGS	encephalo-galeo-synangiosis
EMS	encephalo-myo-synangiosis
EPS	encephalo-pericranium-synangiosis
MBH	multiple burr-hole
MCA	middle cerebral artery
MMD	moyamoya disease
PCA	posterior cerebral artery
STA	superficial temporal artery
TIA	transitory ischemic attack

Author details

Vicente Vanaclocha[1]*, Nieves Saiz-Sapena[2] and Leyre Vanaclocha[3]

1 Department of Surgery, University of Valencia, Valencia, Spain

2 Hospital General Universitario de Valencia, Valencia, Spain

3 Medical School, University College London, London, United Kingdom

*Address all correspondence to: vvanaclo@hotmail.com

References

[1] Takeuchi, K & Shimizu, K. Hypoplasia of the bilateral internal carotid arteries. *Brain Nerve* **9**, 37-43 (1957).

[2] Suzuki, J. & Takaku, A. Cerebrovascular 'moyamoya' disease. Disease showing abnormal net-like vessels in base of brain. *Arch. Neurol.* **20**, 288-299 (1969).

[3] Scott, R. M. & Smith, E. R. Moyamoya disease and moyamoya syndrome. *N. Engl. J. Med.* **360**, 1226-1237 (2009).

[4] Ikeda, E. Systemic vascular changes in spontaneous occlusion of the circle of Willis. *Stroke* **22**, 1358-1362 (1991).

[5] Zhang, Q. *et al.* Clinical Features and Surgical Outcomes of Patients With Moyamoya Disease and the Homozygous RNF213 p.R4810K Variant. *J. Child Neurol.* **34**, 793-800 (2019).

[6] Kim, J. H., Kwon, T.-H., Kim, J. H., Chong, K. & Yoon, W. Intracranial Aneurysms in Adult Moyamoya Disease. *World Neurosurg.* **109**, e175–e182 (2018).

[7] Bang, O. Y., Fujimura, M. & Kim, S.-K. The Pathophysiology of Moyamoya Disease: An Update. *J. Stroke* **18**, 12-20 (2016).

[8] Ogawa, A., Yoshimoto, T., Suzuki, J. & Sakurai, Y. Cerebral blood flow in moyamoya disease. Part 1: Correlation with age and regional distribution. *Acta Neurochir. (Wien)* **105**, 30-34 (1990).

[9] Kawaguchi, S., Sakaki, T., Morimoto, T., Kakizaki, T. & Kamada, K. Characteristics of intracranial aneurysms associated with moyamoya disease. A review of 111 cases. *Acta Neurochir. (Wien)* **138**, 1287-1294 (1996).

[10] Liu, P. *et al.* Intracranial Aneurysms Associated with Moyamoya Disease in Children: Clinical Features and Long-Term Surgical Outcome. *World Neurosurg.* **94**, 513-520 (2016).

[11] Ni, W. *et al.* Treatment of aneurysms in patients with moyamoya disease: a 10-year single-center experience. *J. Neurosurg.* **128**, 1813-1822 (2018).

[12] Ge, P. *et al.* Clinical features, surgical treatment, and outcome of intracranial aneurysms associated with moyamoya disease. *J. Clin. Neurosci. Off. J. Neurosurg. Soc. Australas.* **80**, 274-279 (2020).

[13] Takahashi, J. C. & Miyamoto, S. Moyamoya disease: recent progress and outlook. *Neurol. Med. Chir. (Tokyo)* **50**, 824-832 (2010).

[14] Bhattacharjee, A. K., Tamaki, N., Minami, H. & Ehara, K. Moyamoya disease associated with basilar tip aneurysm. *J. Clin. Neurosci. Off. J. Neurosurg. Soc. Australas.* **6**, 268-271 (1999).

[15] Chen, Y. *et al.* Endovascular Treatment of Ruptured Large or Wide-Neck Basilar Tip Aneurysms Associated with Moyamoya Disease Using the Stent-Assisted Coil Technique. *J. Stroke Cerebrovasc. Dis. Off. J. Natl. Stroke Assoc.* **24**, 2229-2235 (2015).

[16] Furtado, S. V., Medress, Z. A., Teo, M. & Steinberg, G. K. Pathogenesis of aneurysms on major vessels in moyamoya disease and management outcome. *J. Clin. Neurosci. Off. J. Neurosurg. Soc. Australas.* **61**, 219-224 (2019).

[17] Kim, S. *et al.* Clinical Features and Outcomes of Intracranial Aneurysm Associated with Moyamoya Disease. *J. Clin. Neurol. Seoul Korea* **16**, 624-632 (2020).

[18] He, K., Zhu, W., Chen, L. & Mao, Y. Management of distal choroidal artery

aneurysms in patients with moyamoya disease: report of three cases and review of the literature. *World J. Surg. Oncol.* **11**, 187 (2013).

[19] Ni, W. *et al.* Disappearance of aneurysms associated with moyamoya disease after STA-MCA anastomosis with encephaloduro myosynangiosis. *J. Clin. Neurosci. Off. J. Neurosurg. Soc. Australas.* **19**, 485-487 (2012).

[20] Kanamori, F., Takasu, S., Ota, S. & Seki, Y. Prevention of the Rerupture of Collateral Artery Aneurysms on the Ventricular Wall by Early Surgical Revascularization in Moyamoya Disease: Report of Two Cases and Review of the Literature. *World Neurosurg.* **109**, 393-397 (2018).

[21] Kuroda, S., Houkin, K., Kamiyama, H. & Abe, H. Effects of surgical revascularization on peripheral artery aneurysms in moyamoya disease: report of three cases. *Neurosurgery* **49**, 463-467; discussion 467-468 (2001).

[22] Irikura, K. *et al.* The effect of encephalo-myo-synangiosis on abnormal collateral vessels in childhood moyamoya disease. *Neurol. Res.* **22**, 341-346 (2000).

[23] Kodama, N., Sato, M. & Sasaki, T. Treatment of ruptured cerebral aneurysm in moyamoya disease. *Surg. Neurol.* **46**, 62-66 (1996).

[24] Zhao, X., Wang, X., Wang, M., Meng, Q. & Wang, C. Treatment strategies of ruptured intracranial aneurysms associated with moyamoya disease. *Br. J. Neurosurg.* 1-7 (2020) doi:10.1080/02688697.2020.1781058.

[25] See, A. P. *et al.* Down syndrome and moyamoya: clinical presentation and surgical management. *J. Neurosurg. Pediatr.* **16**, 58-63 (2015).

[26] Kauv, P. *et al.* Characteristics of Moyamoya Syndrome in Sickle-Cell Disease by Magnetic Resonance Angiography: An Adult-Cohort Study. *Front. Neurol.* **10**, 15 (2019).

[27] Santoro, C. *et al.* Moyamoya syndrome in children with neurofibromatosis type 1: Italian-French experience. *Am. J. Med. Genet. A.* **173**, 1521-1530 (2017).

[28] Das, S. *et al.* Thalassemia and Moyamoya syndrome: unfurling an intriguing association. *J. Neurol.* **266**, 2838-2847 (2019).

[29] Ni, J. *et al.* Moyamoya syndrome associated with Graves' disease: a case series study. *Ann. Transl. Med.* **2**, 77 (2014).

[30] Scala, M. *et al.* Radiation-Induced Moyamoya Syndrome in Children with Brain Tumors: Case Series and Literature Review. *World Neurosurg.* **135**, 118-129 (2020).

[31] Nariai, T. *et al.* Surgically induced angiogenesis to compensate for hemodynamic cerebral ischemia. *Stroke* **25**, 1014-1021 (1994).

[32] Yamamoto, S. *et al.* Development of Hemorrhage-prone Anastomoses in Asymptomatic Moyamoya Disease-A Comparative Study with Japan Adult Moyamoya Trial. *J. Stroke Cerebrovasc. Dis. Off. J. Natl. Stroke Assoc.* **28**, 104328 (2019).

[33] Schmiedek, P., Piepgras, A., Leinsinger, G., Kirsch, C. M. & Einhüpl, K. Improvement of cerebrovascular reserve capacity by EC-IC arterial bypass surgery in patients with ICA occlusion and hemodynamic cerebral ischemia. *J. Neurosurg.* **81**, 236-244 (1994).

[34] Czabanka, M. *et al.* Characterization of direct and indirect cerebral revascularization for the treatment of European patients with moyamoya disease. *Cerebrovasc. Dis. Basel Switz.* **32**, 361-369 (2011).

[35] Arai, N. *et al.* Hemodynamic stress distribution identified by SPECT reflects ischemic symptoms of Moyamoya disease patients. *Neurosurg. Rev.* **43**, 1323-1329 (2020).

[36] Kim, J. E. & Jeon, J. S. An update on the diagnosis and treatment of adult Moyamoya disease taking into consideration controversial issues. *Neurol. Res.* **36**, 407-416 (2014).

[37] Kim, T. *et al.* Epidemiology of Moyamoya Disease in Korea: Based on National Health Insurance Service Data. *J. Korean Neurosurg. Soc.* **57**, 390-395 (2015).

[38] Kuriyama, S. *et al.* Prevalence and clinicoepidemiological features of moyamoya disease in Japan: findings from a nationwide epidemiological survey. *Stroke* **39**, 42-47 (2008).

[39] Kim, J. S. Moyamoya Disease: Epidemiology, Clinical Features, and Diagnosis. *J. Stroke* **18**, 2-11 (2016).

[40] Yu, L.-B. *et al.* More Precise Imaging Analysis and Diagnosis of Moyamoya Disease and Moyamoya Syndrome Using High-Resolution Magnetic Resonance Imaging. *World Neurosurg.* **96**, 252-260 (2016).

[41] Hu, P., Sun, J., Jin, Y., Shi, X. & Yang, X. Conventional Computed Tomography and Axial Magnetic Resonance T2-Weighted Imaging of Horizontal Segment of Middle Cerebral Artery in Moyamoya Disease or Syndrome in Adult Patients. *J. Stroke Cerebrovasc. Dis. Off. J. Natl. Stroke Assoc.* **24**, 2555-2560 (2015).

[42] Erickson, D. L. & Koivukangas, J. The treatment of Moyamoya disease by superficial temporal-middle cerebral artery (STA-MCA) anastomosis. *Ann. Clin. Res.* **18 Suppl 47**, 21-24 (1986).

[43] Li, J. *et al.* Imaging of Moyamoya Disease and Moyamoya Syndrome: Current Status. *J. Comput. Assist. Tomogr.* **43**, 257-263 (2019).

[44] McAuley, D. J., Poskitt, K. & Steinbok, P. Predicting stroke risk in pediatric moyamoya disease with xenon-enhanced computed tomography. *Neurosurgery* **55**, 327-332; discussion 332-333 (2004).

[45] Wong, T. H., Shagera, Q. A., Ryoo, H. G., Ha, S. & Lee, D. S. Basal and Acetazolamide Brain Perfusion SPECT in Internal Carotid Artery Stenosis. *Nucl. Med. Mol. Imaging* **54**, 9-27 (2020).

[46] Eicker, S. O., Turowski, B., Heiroth, H.-J., Steiger, H.-J. & Hänggi, D. A comparative study of perfusion CT and 99m Tc-HMPAO SPECT measurement to assess cerebrovascular reserve capacity in patients with internal carotid artery occlusion. *Eur. J. Med. Res.* **16**, 484-490 (2011).

[47] Zhang, J. *et al.* Comparative study of MR mTI-ASL and DSC-PWI in evaluating cerebral hemodynamics of patients with Moyamoya disease. *Medicine (Baltimore)* **97**, e12768 (2018).

[48] Hara, S. *et al.* Bayesian Estimation of CBF Measured by DSC-MRI in Patients with Moyamoya Disease: Comparison with 15O-Gas PET and Singular Value Decomposition. *AJNR Am. J. Neuroradiol.* **40**, 1894-1900 (2019).

[49] Pan, H. *et al.* Clinical Prediction of Surgical Revascularization Outcome in Moyamoya Disease Via Transcranial Color Sonography. *J. Stroke Cerebrovasc. Dis. Off. J. Natl. Stroke Assoc.* **29**, 105154 (2020).

[50] Seo, W.-K., Choi, C.-W., Kim, C. K. & Oh, K. Contrast-Enhanced Color-Coded Doppler Sonography in Moyamoya Disease: A Retrospective Study. *Ultrasound Med. Biol.* **44**, 1281-1285 (2018).

[51] Tanaka, K. *et al.* Ultrasonic evaluation of superficial temporal artery-middle cerebral artery anastomosis. *Stroke* **12**, 803-807 (1981).

[52] Baba, T., Houkin, K. & Kuroda, S. Novel epidemiological features of moyamoya disease. *J. Neurol. Neurosurg. Psychiatry* **79**, 900-904 (2008).

[53] Kuroda, S. & Houkin, K. Moyamoya disease: current concepts and future perspectives. *Lancet Neurol.* **7**, 1056-1066 (2008).

[54] Zach, V., Bezov, D., Lipton, R. B. & Ashina, S. Headache associated with moyamoya disease: a case story and literature review. *J. Headache Pain* **11**, 79-82 (2010).

[55] Mikami, T. *et al.* Predictive factors for epilepsy in moyamoya disease. *J. Stroke Cerebrovasc. Dis. Off. J. Natl. Stroke Assoc.* **24**, 17-23 (2015).

[56] Ahn, E. S., Scott, R. M., Robertson, R. L. & Smith, E. R. Chorea in the clinical presentation of moyamoya disease: results of surgical revascularization and a proposed clinicopathological correlation. *J. Neurosurg. Pediatr.* **11**, 313-319 (2013).

[57] Kazumata, K. *et al.* Chronic ischemia alters brain microstructural integrity and cognitive performance in adult moyamoya disease. *Stroke* **46**, 354-360 (2015).

[58] Hirano, Y. *et al.* Association Between the Onset Pattern of Adult Moyamoya Disease and Risk Factors for Stroke. *Stroke* **51**, 3124-3128 (2020).

[59] Duan, L. *et al.* Moyamoya disease in China: its clinical features and outcomes. *Stroke* **43**, 56-60 (2012).

[60] Huang, Z. *et al.* Clinical features and outcomes in 154 patients with haemorrhagic moyamoya disease: comparison of conservative treatment and surgical revascularization. *Neurol. Res.* **37**, 886-892 (2015).

[61] Morioka, M. *et al.* High-risk age for rebleeding in patients with hemorrhagic moyamoya disease: long-term follow-up study. *Neurosurgery* **52**, 1049-1054; discussion 1054-1055 (2003).

[62] Bao, X.-Y. *et al.* Clinical features, surgical treatment, and long-term outcome in pediatric patients with moyamoya disease in China. *Cerebrovasc. Dis. Basel Switz.* **39**, 75-81 (2015).

[63] Kim, K. M. *et al.* Natural History and Risk Factor of Recurrent Hemorrhage in Hemorrhagic Adult Moyamoya Disease. *Neurosurgery* **81**, 289-296 (2017).

[64] Cho, W.-S. *et al.* The natural clinical course of hemodynamically stable adult moyamoya disease. *J. Neurosurg.* **122**, 82-89 (2015).

[65] Li, J. *et al.* Cognitive Performance Profile in Pediatric Moyamoya Disease Patients and Its Relationship With Regional Cerebral Blood Perfusion. *Front. Neurol.* **10**, 1308 (2019).

[66] Kazumata, K. *et al.* Association of cognitive function with cerebral blood flow in children with moyamoya disease. *J. Neurosurg. Pediatr.* 1-7 (2019) doi:10.3171/2019.7.PEDS19312.

[67] Hsu, Y.-H., Kuo, M.-F., Hua, M.-S. & Yang, C.-C. Selective neuropsychological impairments and related clinical factors in children with moyamoya disease of the transient ischemic attack type. *Childs Nerv. Syst. ChNS Off. J. Int. Soc. Pediatr. Neurosurg.* **30**, 441-447 (2014).

[68] Lee, J. Y. *et al.* Delayed posterior circulation insufficiency in pediatric moyamoya disease. *J. Neurol.* **261**, 2305-2313 (2014).

[69] Kimiwada, T., Hayashi, T., Shirane, R. & Tominaga, T. Posterior cerebral artery stenosis and posterior circulation revascularization surgery in pediatric patients with moyamoya disease. *J. Neurosurg. Pediatr.* **21**, 632-638 (2018).

[70] Ge, P. *et al.* Clinical Features of Hemorrhagic Moyamoya Disease in China. *World Neurosurg.* **106**, 224-230 (2017).

[71] Research Committee on the Pathology and Treatment of Spontaneous Occlusion of the Circle of Willis & Health Labour Sciences Research Grant for Research on Measures for Intractable Diseases. Guidelines for diagnosis and treatment of moyamoya disease (spontaneous occlusion of the circle of Willis). *Neurol. Med. Chir. (Tokyo)* **52**, 245-266 (2012).

[72] Kuroda, S. *et al.* Incidence and clinical features of disease progression in adult moyamoya disease. *Stroke* **36**, 2148-2153 (2005).

[73] Chiu, D., Shedden, P., Bratina, P. & Grotta, J. C. Clinical features of moyamoya disease in the United States. *Stroke* **29**, 1347-1351 (1998).

[74] Goyal, M. S. *et al.* Clinical features and outcome in North American adults with idiopathic basal arterial occlusive disease without moyamoya collaterals. *Neurosurgery* **67**, 278-285 (2010).

[75] Starke, R. M. *et al.* Clinical features, surgical treatment, and long-term outcome in adult patients with moyamoya disease. Clinical article. *J. Neurosurg.* **111**, 936-942 (2009).

[76] Miyamoto, S. *et al.* Study of the posterior circulation in moyamoya disease. Clinical and neuroradiological evaluation. *J. Neurosurg.* **61**, 1032-1037 (1984).

[77] Kuroda, S., Ishikawa, T., Houkin, K. & Iwasaki, Y. [Clinical significance of posterior cerebral artery stenosis/occlusion in moyamoya disease]. *No Shinkei Geka.* **30**, 1295-1300 (2002).

[78] Mugikura, S. *et al.* The relationship between cerebral infarction and angiographic characteristics in childhood moyamoya disease. *AJNR Am. J. Neuroradiol.* **20**, 336-343 (1999).

[79] Hishikawa, T., Tokunaga, K., Sugiu, K. & Date, I. Assessment of the difference in posterior circulation involvement between pediatric and adult patients with moyamoya disease. *J. Neurosurg.* **119**, 961-965 (2013).

[80] Funaki, T. *et al.* Angiographic features of hemorrhagic moyamoya disease with high recurrence risk: a supplementary analysis of the Japan Adult Moyamoya Trial. *J. Neurosurg.* **128**, 777-784 (2018).

[81] Ohtoh, T. *et al.* Hemodynamic characteristics of the vertebrobasilar system in moyamoya disease: a histometric study. *Hum. Pathol.* **19**, 465-470 (1988).

[82] Funaki, T. *et al.* High rebleeding risk associated with choroidal collateral vessels in hemorrhagic moyamoya disease: analysis of a nonsurgical cohort in the Japan Adult Moyamoya Trial. *J. Neurosurg.* **130**, 337-673 (2019).

[83] Yamamoto, S. *et al.* Longitudinal anterior-to-posterior shift of collateral channels in patients with moyamoya disease: an implication for its hemorrhagic onset. *J. Neurosurg.* **130**, 884-890 (2018).

[84] Irikura, K. *et al.* A source of haemorrhage in adult patients with moyamoya disease: the significance of tributaries from the choroidal artery. *Acta Neurochir. (Wien)* **138**, 1282-1286 (1996).

[85] Takahashi, J. C. *et al.* Significance of the Hemorrhagic Site for Recurrent

Bleeding: Prespecified Analysis in the Japan Adult Moyamoya Trial. *Stroke* **47**, 37-43 (2016).

[86] Funaki, T. *et al.* Impact of posterior cerebral artery involvement on long-term clinical and social outcome of pediatric moyamoya disease. *J. Neurosurg. Pediatr.* **12**, 626-632 (2013).

[87] Kikuta, K.-I. *et al.* Asymptomatic microbleeds in moyamoya disease: T2*-weighted gradient-echo magnetic resonance imaging study. *J. Neurosurg.* **102**, 470-475 (2005).

[88] Kazumata, K. *et al.* Spatial relationship between cerebral microbleeds, moyamoya vessels, and hematoma in moyamoya disease. *J. Stroke Cerebrovasc. Dis. Off. J. Natl. Stroke Assoc.* **23**, 1421-1428 (2014).

[89] Kuroda, S., Kashiwazaki, D., Ishikawa, T., Nakayama, N. & Houkin, K. Incidence, locations, and longitudinal course of silent microbleeds in moyamoya disease: a prospective T2*-weighted MRI study. *Stroke* **44**, 516-518 (2013).

[90] Schrag, M. & Greer, D. M. Clinical associations of cerebral microbleeds on magnetic resonance neuroimaging. *J. Stroke Cerebrovasc. Dis. Off. J. Natl. Stroke Assoc.* **23**, 2489-2497 (2014).

[91] Sun, W. *et al.* Asymptomatic cerebral microbleeds in adult patients with moyamoya disease: a prospective cohort study with 2 years of follow-up. *Cerebrovasc. Dis. Basel Switz.* **35**, 469-475 (2013).

[92] Yamashita, M., Oka, K. & Tanaka, K. Histopathology of the brain vascular network in moyamoya disease. *Stroke* **14**, 50-58 (1983).

[93] Kikuta, K. *et al.* The presence of multiple microbleeds as a predictor of subsequent cerebral hemorrhage in patients with moyamoya disease. *Neurosurgery* **62**, 104-111, discussion 111-112 (2008).

[94] Qin, Y. *et al.* High incidence of asymptomatic cerebral microbleeds in patients with hemorrhagic onset-type moyamoya disease: a phase-sensitive MRI study and meta-analysis. *Acta Radiol. Stockh. Swed. 1987* **56**, 329-338 (2015).

[95] Kuroda, S., Hashimoto, N., Yoshimoto, T., Iwasaki, Y., & Research Committee on Moyamoya Disease in Japan. Radiological findings, clinical course, and outcome in asymptomatic moyamoya disease: results of multicenter survey in Japan. *Stroke* **38**, 1430-1435 (2007).

[96] Lin, N. *et al.* Discovery of asymptomatic moyamoya arteriopathy in pediatric syndromic populations: radiographic and clinical progression. *Neurosurg. Focus* **31**, E6 (2011).

[97] Yang, J. *et al.* Clinicoepidemiological features of asymptomatic moyamoya disease in adult patients. *J. Cerebrovasc. Endovasc. Neurosurg.* **16**, 241-246 (2014).

[98] He, S. *et al.* Characteristics of cognitive impairment in adult asymptomatic moyamoya disease. *BMC Neurol.* **20**, 322 (2020).

[99] Appireddy, R. *et al.* Surgery for Moyamoya Disease in Children. *J. Child Neurol.* **34**, 517-529 (2019).

[100] Ezura, M. *et al.* Clinical and angiographic follow-up of childhood-onset moyamoya disease. *Childs Nerv. Syst. ChNS Off. J. Int. Soc. Pediatr. Neurosurg.* **11**, 591-594 (1995).

[101] Kelly, M. E., Bell-Stephens, T. E., Marks, M. P., Do, H. M. & Steinberg, G. K. Progression of unilateral moyamoya disease: A clinical series. *Cerebrovasc. Dis. Basel Switz.* **22**, 109-115 (2006).

[102] Yeon, J. Y. *et al.* The prediction of contralateral progression in children

and adolescents with unilateral moyamoya disease. *Stroke* **42**, 2973-2976 (2011).

[103] Luo, R., Gao, F., Deng, X., Zhang, D. & Zhang, Y. Results of Conservative Follow-up or Surgical Treatment of Moyamoya Patients Who Present without Hemorrhage, Transient Ischemic Attack, or Stroke. *World Neurosurg.* **108**, 683-689 (2017).

[104] Fung, L.-W. E., Thompson, D. & Ganesan, V. Revascularisation surgery for paediatric moyamoya: a review of the literature. *Childs Nerv. Syst. ChNS Off. J. Int. Soc. Pediatr. Neurosurg.* **21**, 358-364 (2005).

[105] Hallemeier, C. L. *et al.* Clinical features and outcome in North American adults with moyamoya phenomenon. *Stroke* **37**, 1490-1496 (2006).

[106] Choi, J. U., Kim, D. S., Kim, E. Y. & Lee, K. C. Natural history of moyamoya disease: comparison of activity of daily living in surgery and non surgery groups. *Clin. Neurol. Neurosurg.* **99 Suppl 2**, S11-18 (1997).

[107] Kurokawa, T. *et al.* Prognosis of occlusive disease of the circle of Willis (moyamoya disease) in children. *Pediatr. Neurol.* **1**, 274-277 (1985).

[108] Ng, J., Thompson, D., Lumley, J. P. S., Saunders, D. E. & Ganesan, V. Surgical revascularisation for childhood moyamoya. *Childs Nerv. Syst. ChNS Off. J. Int. Soc. Pediatr. Neurosurg.* **28**, 1041-1048 (2012).

[109] Shang, S. *et al.* Progress in moyamoya disease. *Neurosurg. Rev.* **43**, 371-382 (2020).

[110] Khan, N. *et al.* Failure of primary percutaneous angioplasty and stenting in the prevention of ischemia in Moyamoya angiopathy. *Cerebrovasc. Dis. Basel Switz.* **31**, 147-153 (2011).

[111] Gross, B. A., Thomas, A. J. & Frerichs, K. U. Endovascular treatment of symptomatic moyamoya. *Neurosurg. Rev.* **37**, 579-583 (2014).

[112] Natarajan, S. K. *et al.* Endovascular treatment of patients with intracranial stenosis with moyamoya-type collaterals. *J. Neurointerventional Surg.* **3**, 369-374 (2011).

[113] Houkin, K., Kamiyama, H., Abe, H., Takahashi, A. & Kuroda, S. Surgical therapy for adult moyamoya disease. Can surgical revascularization prevent the recurrence of intracerebral hemorrhage? *Stroke* **27**, 1342-1346 (1996).

[114] Li, Y. *et al.* Surgical treatment of adult moyamoya disease with combined STA-MCA bypass and EDAS: demonstration of technique in video presentation. *Turk. Neurosurg.* **25**, 126-131 (2015).

[115] Miyamoto, S. *et al.* Effects of extracranial-intracranial bypass for patients with hemorrhagic moyamoya disease: results of the Japan Adult Moyamoya Trial. *Stroke* **45**, 1415-1421 (2014).

[116] Li, Q. *et al.* Meta-Analysis of Prognosis of Different Treatments for Symptomatic Moyamoya Disease. *World Neurosurg.* **127**, 354-361 (2019).

[117] Porras, J. L. *et al.* Effectiveness of Ipsilateral Stroke Prevention Between Conservative Management and Indirect Revascularization for Moyamoya Disease in a North American Cohort. *World Neurosurg.* **110**, e928–e936 (2018).

[118] Kawaguchi, S., Okuno, S. & Sakaki, T. Effect of direct arterial bypass on the prevention of future stroke in patients with the hemorrhagic variety of moyamoya disease. *J. Neurosurg.* **93**, 397-401 (2000).

[119] Kuroda, S., Houkin, K., Ishikawa, T., Nakayama, N. & Iwasaki, Y. Novel

bypass surgery for moyamoya disease using pericranial flap: its impacts on cerebral hemodynamics and long-term outcome. *Neurosurgery* **66**, 1093-1101; discussion 1101 (2010).

[120] Miyamoto, S. *et al.* Long-term outcome after STA-MCA anastomosis for moyamoya disease. *Neurosurg. Focus* **5**, e5 (1998).

[121] Jeon, J. P. *et al.* Meta-analysis of the surgical outcomes of symptomatic moyamoya disease in adults. *J. Neurosurg.* **128**, 793-799 (2018).

[122] Gupta, R. *et al.* Clinical presentation, progression, and treatment outcomes of moyamoya disease in the elderly. *Acta Neurochir. (Wien)* **158**, 2409-2414 (2016).

[123] Karasawa, J., Kikuchi, H., Furuse, S., Kawamura, J. & Sakaki, T. Treatment of moyamoya disease with STA-MCA anastomosis. *J. Neurosurg.* **49**, 679-688 (1978).

[124] Kazumata, K. *et al.* Direct Anastomosis Using Occipital Artery for Additional Revascularization in Moyamoya Disease After Combined Superficial Temporal Artery-Middle Cerebral Artery and Indirect Bypass. *Oper. Neurosurg. Hagerstown Md* **13**, 213-223 (2017).

[125] Yokoya, S., Hino, A., Goto, Y. & Oka, H. Middle Meningeal-Middle Cerebral Artery Anastomosis for Moyamoya Disease. *World Neurosurg.* **129**, 5-8 (2019).

[126] Hendricks, B. K. & Spetzler, R. F. Moyamoya Disease Superficial Temporal Artery-to-Middle Cerebral Artery Onlay: 2-Dimensional Operative Video. *Oper. Neurosurg. Hagerstown Md* **18**, E229 (2020).

[127] Iwama, T., Hashimoto, N., Tsukahara, T. & Miyake, H. Superficial temporal artery to anterior cerebral artery direct anastomosis in patients with moyamoya disease. *Clin. Neurol. Neurosurg.* **99 Suppl 2**, S134-136 (1997).

[128] Hayashi, T., Shirane, R. & Tominaga, T. Additional surgery for postoperative ischemic symptoms in patients with moyamoya disease: the effectiveness of occipital artery-posterior cerebral artery bypass with an indirect procedure: technical case report. *Neurosurgery* **64**, E195-196; discussion E196 (2009).

[129] Hirano, T. *et al.* Occipital Artery to Middle Cerebral Artery Bypass in Cases of Unavailable Superficial Temporal Artery. *World Neurosurg.* **112**, 101-108 (2018).

[130] Lee, M., Guzman, R., Bell-Stephens, T. & Steinberg, G. K. Intraoperative blood flow analysis of direct revascularization procedures in patients with moyamoya disease. *J. Cereb. Blood Flow Metab. Off. J. Int. Soc. Cereb. Blood Flow Metab.* **31**, 262-274 (2011).

[131] Veeravagu, A. *et al.* Moyamoya disease in pediatric patients: outcomes of neurosurgical interventions. *Neurosurg. Focus* **24**, E16 (2008).

[132] Ahn, J. H. *et al.* Hemorrhagic moyamoya disease in children: clinical features and surgical outcome. *Childs Nerv. Syst. ChNS Off. J. Int. Soc. Pediatr. Neurosurg.* **28**, 237-245 (2012).

[133] Hayashi, T., Shirane, R., Fujimura, M. & Tominaga, T. Postoperative neurological deterioration in pediatric moyamoya disease: watershed shift and hyperperfusion. *J. Neurosurg. Pediatr.* **6**, 73-81 (2010).

[134] Chen, Y. *et al.* Postoperative hemorrhage during the acute phase after direct or combined revascularization for moyamoya disease: risk factors, prognosis, and literature review.

J. Neurosurg. 1-10 (2019) doi:10.3171/2019.7.JNS19885.

[135] Fujimura, M. *et al.* Efficacy of prophylactic blood pressure lowering according to a standardized postoperative management protocol to prevent symptomatic cerebral hyperperfusion after direct revascularization surgery for moyamoya disease. *Cerebrovasc. Dis. Basel Switz.* **33**, 436-445 (2012).

[136] Guzman, R. *et al.* Clinical outcome after 450 revascularization procedures for moyamoya disease. Clinical article. *J. Neurosurg.* **111**, 927-935 (2009).

[137] Egashira, Y. *et al.* Disruption of Cortical Arterial Network is Associated with the Severity of Transient Neurologic Events After Direct Bypass Surgery in Adult Moyamoya Disease. *World Neurosurg.* **100**, 311-315 (2017).

[138] Suzuki, H. *et al.* Assessment of the cortical artery using computed tomography angiography for bypass surgery in moyamoya disease. *Neurosurg. Rev.* **40**, 299-307 (2017).

[139] Houkin, K., Kuroda, S., Ishikawa, T. & Abe, H. Neovascularization (angiogenesis) after revascularization in moyamoya disease. Which technique is most useful for moyamoya disease? *Acta Neurochir. (Wien)* **142**, 269-276 (2000).

[140] Chou, S.-C. *et al.* Improving Indirect Revascularization for Effective Treatment of Adult Moyamoya Disease: A Prospective Clinical, Cerebral Angiographic, and Perfusion Study. *World Neurosurg.* **119**, e180–e191 (2018).

[141] Imai, H. *et al.* The importance of encephalo-myo-synangiosis in surgical revascularization strategies for moyamoya disease in children and adults. *World Neurosurg.* **83**, 691-699 (2015).

[142] Karasawa, J., Kikuchi, H., Furuse, S., Sakaki, T. & Yoshida, Y. A surgical treatment of 'moyamoya' disease 'encephalo-myo synangiosis'. *Neurol. Med. Chir. (Tokyo)* **17**, 29-37 (1977).

[143] Gadgil, N. *et al.* Indirect revascularization with the dural inversion technique for pediatric moyamoya disease: 20-year experience. *J. Neurosurg. Pediatr.* **22**, 541-549 (2018).

[144] Kashiwagi, S. *et al.* Revascularization with split duro-encephalo-synangiosis in the pediatric moyamoya disease--surgical result and clinical outcome. *Clin. Neurol. Neurosurg.* **99 Suppl 2**, S115-117 (1997).

[145] Kashiwagi, S. *et al.* Use of a split dura for revascularization of ischemic hemispheres in moyamoya disease. *J. Neurosurg.* **85**, 380-383 (1996).

[146] Shen, W. *et al.* Enlarged Encephalo-Duro-Myo-Synangiosis Treatment for Moyamoya Disease in Young Children. *World Neurosurg.* **106**, 9-16 (2017).

[147] Kuroda, S. *et al.* Late (5-20 years) outcomes after STA-MCA anastomosis and encephalo-duro-myo-arterio-pericranial synangiosis in patients with moyamoya disease. *J. Neurosurg.* 1-8 (2020) doi:10.3171/2019.12.JNS192938.

[148] Byun, Y. H. *et al.* Preservation of the Arachnoid Membrane During Encephaloduroarteriosynangiosis Reduces Postoperative Complications without Undermining the Surgical Outcome in Pediatric Moyamoya Disease. *World Neurosurg.* **130**, e406–e416 (2019).

[149] Park, J. H. *et al.* Modified encephaloduroarteriosynangiosis with bifrontal encephalogaleoperiosteal synangiosis for the treatment of pediatric moyamoya disease. Technical note. *J. Neurosurg.* **106**, 237-242 (2007).

[150] Kim, S.-K., Wang, K.-C., Kim, I.-O., Lee, D. S. & Cho, B.-K. Combined

encephaloduroarteriosynangiosis and bifrontal encephalogaleo (periosteal) synangiosis in pediatric moyamoya disease. *Neurosurgery* **62**, 1456-1464 (2008).

[151] Kalra, N., Bautista, M., McCullagh, H. & Tyagi, A. PedsQL Score Post Encephalo-duro-arterio-myo-synangiosis Procedure for Moyamoya Disease: A Single Center Experience. *World Neurosurg.* **144**, e674–e678 (2020).

[152] Ogiwara, H. & Morota, N. Bifrontal encephalogaleosynangiosis for children with moyamoya disease. *J. Neurosurg. Pediatr.* **10**, 246-251 (2012).

[153] Kim, C.-Y. *et al.* Encephaloduroarteriosynangiosis with bifrontal encephalogaleo(periosteal) synangiosis in the pediatric moyamoya disease: the surgical technique and its outcomes. *Childs Nerv. Syst. ChNS Off. J. Int. Soc. Pediatr. Neurosurg.* **19**, 316-324 (2003).

[154] Zhao, Y. *et al.* Modified encephalo-duro-periosteal-synangiosis (EDPS) for the revascularization of anterior cerebral artery territory in moyamoya disease: A single-center experience. *Clin. Neurol. Neurosurg.* **178**, 86-92 (2019).

[155] Li, W. *et al.* Complications of contralateral C-7 transfer through the modified prespinal route for repairing brachial plexus root avulsion injury: a retrospective study of 425 patients. *J. Neurosurg.* **122**, 1421-1428 (2015).

[156] Karasawa, J., Kikuchi, H., Kawamura, J. & Sakai, T. Intracranial transplantation of the omentum for cerebrovascular moyamoya disease: a two-year follow-up study. *Surg. Neurol.* **14**, 444-449 (1980).

[157] Navarro, R. *et al.* Less invasive pedicled omental-cranial transposition in pediatric patients with moyamoya disease and failed prior revascularization. *Neurosurgery* **10 Suppl 1**, 1-14 (2014).

[158] Mirone, G. *et al.* Multiple Burr-Hole Surgery for the Treatment of Moyamoya Disease and Quasi-Moyamoya Disease in Children: Preliminary Surgical and Imaging Results. *World Neurosurg.* **127**, e843–e855 (2019).

[159] Zhao, X., Wang, C., Ji, Y., Han, C. & Wang, M. Therapeutic effect of multiple burr hole operation combined with dural inversion and periosteal synangiosis for moyamoya disease. *Br. J. Neurosurg.* **29**, 811-817 (2015).

[160] McLaughlin, N. & Martin, N. A. Effectiveness of burr holes for indirect revascularization in patients with moyamoya disease-a review of the literature. *World Neurosurg.* **81**, 91-98 (2014).

[161] Kawaguchi, T. *et al.* Multiple burr-hole operation for adult moyamoya disease. *J. Neurosurg.* **84**, 468-476 (1996).

[162] Oliveira, R. S. de *et al.* Effect of multiple cranial burr hole surgery on prevention of recurrent ischemic attacks in children with moyamoya disease. *Neuropediatrics* **40**, 260-264 (2009).

[163] Kazumata, K. *et al.* The frequency of postoperative stroke in moyamoya disease following combined revascularization: a single-university series and systematic review. *J. Neurosurg.* **121**, 432-440 (2014).

[164] Wouters, A., Smets, I., Van den Noortgate, W., Steinberg, G. K. & Lemmens, R. Cerebrovascular events after surgery versus conservative therapy for moyamoya disease: a meta-analysis. *Acta Neurol. Belg.* **119**, 305-313 (2019).

[165] Houkin, K., Nakayama, N., Kuroda, S., Ishikawa, T. & Nonaka, T.

How does angiogenesis develop in pediatric moyamoya disease after surgery? A prospective study with MR angiography. *Childs Nerv. Syst. ChNS Off. J. Int. Soc. Pediatr. Neurosurg.* **20**, 734-741 (2004).

[166] Pandey, P. & Steinberg, G. K. Outcome of repeat revascularization surgery for moyamoya disease after an unsuccessful indirect revascularization. Clinical article. *J. Neurosurg.* **115**, 328-336 (2011).

[167] Cahan, L. D. Failure of encephalo-duro-arterio-synangiosis procedure in moyamoya disease. *Pediatr. Neurosci.* **12**, 58-62 (1985).

[168] Miyamoto, S. *et al.* Pitfalls in the surgical treatment of moyamoya disease. Operative techniques for refractory cases. *J. Neurosurg.* **68**, 537-543 (1988).

[169] Lanterna, L. A. Moyamoya Disease: From Hypoperfusion to Network Disruption. *World Neurosurg.* **104**, 1036-1037 (2017).

[170] Krayenbühl, H. A. The Moyamoya syndrome and the neurosurgeon. *Surg. Neurol.* **4**, 353-360 (1975).

[171] Kikuchi, H & Karasawa, J. STA-cortical MCA anastomosis for cerebrovascular occlusive disease. *No Shinkei Geka.* **1**, 15-19 (1973).

[172] Nakagawa, Y. *et al.* [Reconstructive operation for moyamoya disease. Surgical indication for the hemorrhagic type, and preferable operative methods]. *Neurol. Med. Chir. (Tokyo)* **23**, 464-470 (1983).

[173] Spetzler, R. F., Roski, R. A. & Kopaniky, D. R. Alternative superficial temporal artery to middle cerebral artery revascularization procedure. *Neurosurgery* 7, 484-487 (1980).

[174] Takeuchi, S. *et al.* Treatment of moyamoya disease by temporal muscle graft 'encephalo-myo-synangiosis'. *Childs Brain* **10**, 1-15 (1983).

[175] Matsushima, Y *et al.* A new operative method for 'moyamoya' disease: A presentation of a case who underwent encephalo-duro-arterio(STA)-synangiosis. *Shoni No Noshinkei* **5**, 249-255 (1980).

[176] Matsushima, Y. & Inaba, Y. Moyamoya disease in children and its surgical treatment. Introduction of a new surgical procedure and its follow-up angiograms. *Childs Brain* **11**, 155-170 (1984).

[177] Tenjin, H. & Ueda, S. Multiple EDAS (encephalo-duro-arterio-synangiosis). Additional EDAS using the frontal branch of the superficial temporal artery (STA) and the occipital artery for pediatric moyamoya patients in whom EDAS using the parietal branch of STA was insufficient. *Childs Nerv. Syst. ChNS Off. J. Int. Soc. Pediatr. Neurosurg.* **13**, 220-224 (1997).

[178] Ge, P. *et al.* Encephaloduroarterio synangiosis versus conservative treatment for patients with moyamoya disease at late Suzuki stage. *J. Clin. Neurosci. Off. J. Neurosurg. Soc. Australas.* **50**, 277-280 (2018).

[179] Wang, Q.-N. *et al.* Encephaloduro arteriosynangiosis for hemorrhagic moyamoya disease: long-term outcome of a consecutive series of 95 adult patients from a single center. *J. Neurosurg.* **130**, 1898-1905 (2019).

[180] Ren, B. *et al.* Surgical outcomes following encephaloduroarterio synangiosis in adult moyamoya disease associated with Type 2 diabetes. *J. Neurosurg.* **125**, 308-314 (2016).

[181] Chiarelli, P. A., Patel, A. P., Lee, A., Chandra, S. R. & Sekhar, L. N. Sternocleidomastoid Encephalomyo synangiosis for Treatment-Resistant

Moyamoya Disease. *Oper. Neurosurg. Hagerstown Md* **17**, E23–E28 (2019).

[182] Yoshioka, N., Tominaga, S. & Inui, T. Cerebral revascularization using omentum and serratus anterior muscle free flap transfer for adult moyamoya disease: case report. *Surg. Neurol.* **46**, 430-435; discussion 435-436 (1996).

[183] Touho, H., Karasawa, J. & Ohnishi, H. Cerebral revascularization using gracilis muscle transplantation for childhood moyamoya disease. *Surg. Neurol.* **43**, 191-197; discussion 197-198 (1995).

[184] Yoshioka, N. & Tominaga, S. Cerebral revascularization using latissimus dorsi muscle free flap transfer--technical note. *Neurol. Med. Chir. (Tokyo)* **37**, 288-291 (1997).

[185] Endo, M., Kawano, N., Miyaska, Y. & Yada, K. Cranial burr hole for revascularization in moyamoya disease. *J. Neurosurg.* **71**, 180-185 (1989).

[186] Inoue, T *et al.* Frontal encephalo-myo-arterio-synangiosis (EMAS). *Nosotchu No Geka* **20**, 297-300.

[187] Kinugasa, K. *et al.* Ribbon enchephalo-duro-arterio-myo-synangiosis for moyamoya disease. *Surg. Neurol.* **41**, 455-461 (1994).

[188] Thines, L. *et al.* Surgical management of Moyamoya disease and syndrome: Current concepts and personal experience. *Rev. Neurol. (Paris)* **171**, 31-44 (2015).

[189] Abla, A. A. *et al.* Surgical outcomes for moyamoya angiopathy at barrow neurological institute with comparison of adult indirect encephaloduroarteriosynangiosis bypass, adult direct superficial temporal artery-to-middle cerebral artery bypass, and pediatric bypass: 154 revas cularization surgeries in 140 affected hemispheres. *Neurosurgery* **73**, 430-439 (2013).

[190] Zhao, M. *et al.* Adolescents with moyamoya disease: clinical features, surgical treatment and long-term outcomes. *Acta Neurochir. (Wien)* **159**, 2071-2080 (2017).

[191] King, J. A. J., Armstrong, D., Vachhrajani, S. & Dirks, P. B. Relative contributions of the middle meningeal artery and superficial temporal artery in revascularization surgery for moyamoya syndrome in children: the results of superselective angiography. *J. Neurosurg. Pediatr.* **5**, 184-189 (2010).

[192] Wang, G. *et al.* Membrane Retraction Technique in Bypass Surgery for the Treatment of Adult Moyamoya Disease with Deep-Seated Recipient Artery. *World Neurosurg.* **139**, 294-297 (2020).

[193] Ge, P. *et al.* Postoperative collateral formation after indirect bypass for hemorrhagic moyamoya disease. *BMC Neurol.* **20**, 28 (2020).

[194] Kim, S.-K. *et al.* Pediatric moyamoya disease: An analysis of 410 consecutive cases. *Ann. Neurol.* **68**, 92-101 (2010).

[195] Mizoi, K., Kayama, T., Yoshimoto, T. & Nagamine, Y. Indirect revascularization for moyamoya disease: is there a beneficial effect for adult patients? *Surg. Neurol.* **45**, 541-548; discussion 548-549 (1996).

[196] Kim, T., Oh, C. W., Bang, J. S., Kim, J. E. & Cho, W.-S. Moyamoya Disease: Treatment and Outcomes. *J. Stroke* **18**, 21-30 (2016).

[197] Liu, J. J. & Steinberg, G. K. Direct Versus Indirect Bypass for Moyamoya Disease. *Neurosurg. Clin. N. Am.* **28**, 361-374 (2017).

[198] Feghali, J. *et al.* Differing Surgical Outcomes in a Multiethnic Cohort

Suggest Racial Phenotypes in Moyamoya Disease. *World Neurosurg.* **128**, e865–e872 (2019).

[199] Isono, M. *et al.* Long-term outcomes of pediatric moyamoya disease treated by encephalo-duro-arterio-synangiosis. *Pediatr. Neurosurg.* **36**, 14-21 (2002).

[200] Chen, C., Wang, H., Hou, B., Luo, L. & Guo, Y. Surgical Revascularization for Children with Moyamoya Disease: A New Modification to the Pial Synangiosis. *World Neurosurg.* **110**, e203–e211 (2018).

[201] Touho, H., Karasawa, J., Ohnishi, H., Yamada, K. & Shibamoto, K. Surgical reconstruction of failed indirect anastomosis in childhood Moyamoya disease. *Neurosurgery* **32**, 935-940; discussion 940 (1993).

[202] Piao, J., Wu, W., Yang, Z. & Yu, J. Research Progress of Moyamoya Disease in Children. *Int. J. Med. Sci.* **12**, 566-575 (2015).

[203] Xu, B. *et al.* Superficial temporal artery-middle cerebral artery bypass combined with encephalo-duro-myo-synangiosis in treating moyamoya disease: surgical techniques, indications and midterm follow-up results. *Chin. Med. J. (Engl.)* **125**, 4398-4405 (2012).

[204] Noshiro, S. *et al.* Neuromodulatory Role of Revascularization Surgery in Moyamoya Disease. *World Neurosurg.* **91**, 473-482 (2016).

[205] Deng, X. *et al.* Effects of different surgical modalities on the clinical outcome of patients with moyamoya disease: a prospective cohort study. *J. Neurosurg.* **128**, 1327-1337 (2018).

[206] Ishikawa, T., Houkin, K., Kamiyama, H. & Abe, H. Effects of surgical revascularization on outcome of patients with pediatric moyamoya disease. *Stroke* **28**, 1170-1173 (1997).

[207] Kim, D.-S. *et al.* Surgical treatment of moyamoya disease in adults: combined direct and indirect vs. indirect bypass surgery. *Neurol. Med. Chir. (Tokyo)* **52**, 333-338 (2012).

[208] Czabanka, M., Vajkoczy, P., Schmiedek, P. & Horn, P. Age-dependent revascularization patterns in the treatment of moyamoya disease in a European patient population. *Neurosurg. Focus* **26**, E9 (2009).

[209] Jagdevan, S., Sriganesh, K., Pandey, P., Reddy, M. & Umamaheswara Rao, G. S. Anesthetic factors and outcome in children undergoing indirect revascularization procedure for moyamoya disease: An Indian perspective. *Neurol. India* **63**, 702-706 (2015).

[210] Iwama, T., Hashimoto, N. & Yonekawa, Y. The relevance of hemodynamic factors to perioperative ischemic complications in childhood moyamoya disease. *Neurosurgery* **38**, 1120-1125; discussion 1125-1126 (1996).

[211] Arias, E. J., Derdeyn, C. P., Dacey, R. G. & Zipfel, G. J. Advances and surgical considerations in the treatment of moyamoya disease. *Neurosurgery* **74 Suppl 1**, S116-125 (2014).

[212] Lee, J. K., Williams, M., Reyes, M. & Ahn, E. S. Cerebrovascular blood pressure autoregulation monitoring and postoperative transient ischemic attack in pediatric moyamoya vasculopathy. *Paediatr. Anaesth.* **28**, 94-102 (2018).

[213] Nomura, S. *et al.* Perioperative management protocols for children with moyamoya disease. *Childs Nerv. Syst. ChNS Off. J. Int. Soc. Pediatr. Neurosurg.* **17**, 270-274 (2001).

[214] Schubert, G. A. *et al.* Perfusion characteristics of Moyamoya disease: an anatomically and clinically oriented analysis and comparison. *Stroke* **45**, 101-106 (2014).

[215] Jo, K.-I., Yeon, J. Y., Hong, S.-C. & Kim, J.-S. Clinical course of asymptomatic adult moyamoya disease. *Cerebrovasc. Dis. Basel Switz.* **37**, 94-101 (2014).

[216] Cheung, A. H.-K. *et al.* Surgical Outcome for Moyamoya Disease: Clinical and Perfusion Computed Tomography Correlation. *World Neurosurg.* **98**, 81-88 (2017).

[217] Matsushima, T. *et al.* Reoperation for moyamoya disease refractory to encephalo-duro-arterio-synangiosis. *Acta Neurochir. (Wien)* **107**, 129-132 (1990).

[218] Kim, T. *et al.* Stroke prevention by direct revascularization for patients with adult-onset moyamoya disease presenting with ischemia. *J. Neurosurg.* **124**, 1788-1793 (2016).

[219] Qian, C. *et al.* The Efficacy of Surgical Treatment for the Secondary Prevention of Stroke in Symptomatic Moyamoya Disease: A Meta-Analysis. *Medicine (Baltimore)* **94**, e2218 (2015).

[220] Wang, G., Zhang, X., Feng, M., Liu, X. & Guo, F. Efficacy of Surgical Treatment on the Recurrent Stroke Prevention for Adult Patients With Hemorrhagic Moyamoya Disease. *J. Craniofac. Surg.* **28**, 2113-2116 (2017).

[221] Jang, D.-K. *et al.* Bypass surgery versus medical treatment for symptomatic moyamoya disease in adults. *J. Neurosurg.* **127**, 492-502 (2017).

[222] Fujii, K., Ikezaki, K., Irikura, K., Miyasaka, Y. & Fukui, M. The efficacy of bypass surgery for the patients with hemorrhagic moyamoya disease. *Clin. Neurol. Neurosurg.* **99 Suppl 2**, S194-195 (1997).

[223] Funaki, T. *et al.* Incidence of late cerebrovascular events after direct bypass among children with moyamoya disease: a descriptive longitudinal study at a single center. *Acta Neurochir. (Wien)* **156**, 551-559; discussion 559 (2014).

[224] Cho, W.-S. *et al.* Long-term outcomes after combined revascularization surgery in adult moyamoya disease. *Stroke* **45**, 3025-3031 (2014).

[225] Liu, X. *et al.* Clinical features and long-term outcomes of moyamoya disease: a single-center experience with 528 cases in China. *J. Neurosurg.* **122**, 392-399 (2015).

[226] Starke, R. M., Komotar, R. J. & Connolly, E. S. Optimal surgical treatment for moyamoya disease in adults: direct versus indirect bypass. *Neurosurg. Focus* **26**, E8 (2009).

[227] Funaki, T., Takahashi, J. C. & Miyamoto, S. Late Cerebrovascular Events and Social Outcome after Adolescence: Long-term Outcome of Pediatric Moyamoya Disease. *Neurol. Med. Chir. (Tokyo)* **58**, 240-246 (2018).

[228] Yamao, Y. *et al.* Revascularization Surgery in Childhood Associated with a Low Incidence of Microbleeds in Adult Patients with Moyamoya. *World Neurosurg.* **133**, e716–e721 (2020).

[229] Fiaschi, P. *et al.* Limits and pitfalls of indirect revascularization in moyamoya disease and syndrome. *Neurosurg. Rev.* (4):1877-1887 (2020) doi:10.1007/s10143-020-01393-1.

[230] Macyszyn, L. *et al.* Direct versus indirect revascularization procedures for moyamoya disease: a comparative effectiveness study. *J. Neurosurg.* **126**, 1523-1529 (2017).

[231] Zhai, X. *et al.* Risk Factors Associated with Neurologic Deterioration After Combined Direct and Indirect Revascularization in Patients with Moyamoya Disease on the

East Coast of China. *World Neurosurg.* **118**, e92–e98 (2018).

[232] Hyun, S.-J., Kim, J.-S. & Hong, S.-C. Prognostic factors associated with perioperative ischemic complications in adult-onset moyamoya disease. *Acta Neurochir. (Wien)* **152**, 1181-1188 (2010).

[233] Kim, S.-H., Choi, J.-U., Yang, K.-H., Kim, T.-G. & Kim, D.-S. Risk factors for postoperative ischemic complications in patients with moyamoya disease. *J. Neurosurg.* **103**, 433-438 (2005).

[234] Lee, J. Y. *et al.* Neurocognitive profiles of children with moyamoya disease before and after surgical intervention. *Cerebrovasc. Dis. Basel Switz.* **31**, 230-237 (2011).

[235] Zeng, H. *et al.* Comparison of Operative and Conservative Treatment for Asymptomatic Moyamoya Disease: Preliminary Experience in Small Retrospective Series. *World Neurosurg.* **146**, e955–e960 (2021).